# Colloidal Production Guide Volume II 2009 Update
## Introduction to the Guide

This guide is written specifically for the home or small commercial colloidal producer using the safer, low voltage direct current (lvdc at under 30 vdc and 1 amp) Ionic method. There are also sections which are written towards the more advanced Nano-Particulate production methods using high voltage alternating current (hvac 10-15kv @ 30 ma max) methods.

This book is provided to assist the amateur and/or advanced colloidal producer or researcher in understanding the minimal requirements, methods and even the dangers associated with LVDC and HVAC colloidal production by use of power supplies and lab experiments.

Pride Scientific , Pride Electronic Labs, Pride Communications, Nature's Spirit Colloidal Minerals, the authors and contributors of this guide make no claim as this guides usefulness in creating proper, safe or pristine colloidal minerals for your personal or commercial use. Please be advised that while we have lab tested and checked each experiment from our own safety and use purpose, there are a few experiments contained in this book that have been submitted by fellow Colloidal Researchers and 'lay' scientists that are not accredited professionals. The safety information provided in this document should be interpreted with this distinction clearly in mind. The authors and publishers hereby disclaim any liability for injury to persons or property that may result due to the construction or use of colloidal LVDC through HVAC power supplies. Experiments and ideas presented in this guide cover low through high voltage apparatus.

This Guide is for informational purposes only, and the authors or contributors, nor the publisher make any claims to its usefulness or completeness or accuracy. While many of the dangers associated with the use of using voltage and amperage around a water base have been pointed out in this document, other potential hazards may exist. All power supplies and electrical devices used near or in water batches are inherently dangerous and should only be attempted, constructed and operated by individuals familiar with proper DC/AC safety measures.

## Acknowledgements

**Marc Peterson** is a certified and licensed Electronics Technician with a specialized certificate in Radio Frequency/Electrical design and engineering. He holds several other licensees and certificates in Radio and Audio Technical design. Marc also is Amateur Radio Operator and serves with Emergency Services. He is the Director of the RMRA and is a voting board member of the CSRG. He is responsible for compiling much of the data and research contained in this book. Credit for the book goes out to the many past research partners who have contributed to this latest volume. Marc wishes to thank the many colloidal pioneers who have perfected and revised his original methods he discovered and were published first in 1996. He is also the owner of Pride Scientific and Marc's hobbies include being an airplane pilot, a published author or both written and photographic books, and a musician with 4 mediation albums out this time.

**Dr. Daniel Guthrie** is a Doctor of Chiropractic, who helped me see the value of Alternative Therapies using light, sound and energy, has helped many through alternative medicine.

**Donald Grant** is a very smart and talented Colloidal Researcher who is always ahead of the colloidal production game. Don is always presenting his work and sharing his wonderful knowledge and insights of good colloidal production. His ideas regarding new research in using vacuum argon chamber designs will someday take Colloidal Production to a whole new level.  Don continues to educate and share his knowledge with the Colloidal Research community.

The Guide is set up as pages and sections rather than chapters, as there is so much information on each subject that happens to be interrelated to other sections and experiments. It is most helpful to take the time to read and study each page, because each experiment corroborates each other experiment throughout the guide. Some of the sections seem to duplicate the each other, but if you look read them carefully, there are slight differences required to perfect the mode, method and production to each mineral.

## CONTENTS

For support or free help,
Visit us at:
**Pacific-Organix Labs**
www.pacific-organix.com

## Preface

It is very important that you as the reader take the time to comprehend and fully understand this entire guide, including this section. At this time, the books sections do interrelate and unfortunately jump around from item to item and hopefully in future editions we will only have one method to present. But for right now, there are several methods we will be looking at creating and covering.

Many of the questions about experiments and testing are answered in the section you are working on, however, please feel free to email Pride Scientific at anytime for free assistance.
mfp.pacific@gmail.com

Some experiments are quite dangerous to recreate in your field lab. Pride Scientific and the author(s) assume that you have prior chemistry lab experience and have taken the appropriate AC/DC electronic coursework and know about electrical safety measures and requirements. If you have not, don't despair, we will try and educate you on a few of the small dangers and common mistakes in using lvdc and hvac power supplies.

### PLEASE READ THE SAFETY SECTION BEFORE PROCEEDING OR JUMPING AHEAD IN THIS GUIDE!

The production guide sections of this book contain both IONIC and PARTICULATE colloidal production data; experiments and ideas for the best production. The experiments shown in each section are industry standard methods (and a few others) that will help you accurately produce pristine, safe and effective colloidal mineral liquid supplements for human, animal or plant use.

All of the experiments and information contained in this guide has been tested in laboratory controlled settings and considered safe when using Chemistry and Electronics safety procedures. This guide is for informational purposes only. Pride Scientific, the Author(s) and contributors to these chapters are not liable, civilly or criminally for your misuse of the information contained herein. Please read the Instructional manuals included with your DIGIPRO Colloidal Lab generation equipment (and any safety update addendums) that are included with your system.

Please go to our website and email or call us if you have any production or experiment questions or comments. We want to hear from you even if you want to report a misspelled word in this book (believe me, there are many of them).

Many of the experiments and data listed for each production method has been lab tested by Pride Scientific as well as other prominent University Research team members many thousands of times. Each field researcher or producer who finds a better or easier way of production has been gracious enough to share many of these 'expanded' experiments and methods to add scope to this book. Please feel free to let us know your special tricks as well and we'll add it to the manual (and credit you) for all others to learn about and try out in the field.

This book is published by Amazon-Create Publishing and updated semi-annually. The book is published through Amazon.com and Create on demand. This allows us to make changes, additions and add new methods as we go along. This allows us to keep you, our fellow researcher and producer up-to-date with the changing industry and production techniques.

Throughout this book (or guide as it is referred to allot) we have attempted to provide you with the best information that we know of, so you can produce safe and effective colloidal products. Unfortunately, it may now (or soon will be) unlawful to purchase, posses or make certain colloidal products in your various areas. For instance, there are always new regulations hampering your production attempts. Currently in the USA, there are several new EPA and FDA US regulations attacking colloidal producers and users. The US DSHEA also has strict new product labeling requirements that went in effect in late 2006. You should check your local and federal regulations before buying or making colloidal products.

Some of the actual methods we will discuss in each section are actually of our own work, while other methods are ideas shared by our field research partners and scientific staff is included and credit is given to those researchers where applicable. You will notice that this book does not carry any foot notes, technical links or other individual citations; this is because about 99% of the methods and procedures written in this book are actual original idea and production methods discovered by Pride Scientific beginning in 1996. All of the methods that are discussed in this latest volume are published with the permission and authorization of the methods individual author, owner or patent holders. To make colloidal minerals, you should seek out or make available a clean lab setting or area, preferably an office or minimally special clean area for colloidal production. It also helps to buy the correct colloidal generation equipment and lab-ware supplies. This is where Pride Scientific will really help you get going.

Besides Pride Scientific DIGIPRO colloidal generation systems, there are several good quality suppliers of production equipment out there. This guide covers basic through advanced production techniques and setting requirements that only the wide range DIGIPRO systems can be set to, however, we have included 'close' settings of current and voltage settings that will effectively allow you to use ANY colloidal power supply system to produce decent colloidal minerals.

Once you have your basic lab set up with the proper equipment installed, you should be able to recreate our methods and produce quality colloidal products. It is important that you follow the experiment steps and try not to short cut or deviate from the production method instructions. We have about 50% of new users complain to us that they are *ruining* their batches of colloidal minerals, only to find out that they skipped around and went into the production section without reading the 'HOW's or WHY's' behind the experiment.

For instance, if you are using any NST (neon sign transformer) to make HVAC Colloidal Gold, you must use our PUAM (plasma underwater arc method) which is the only way to produce pink or reddish tinted, colloidal Nano Gold at this time. One of the by-products of using the PUAM is that it acts like a powerful radio transmitter while running. This transmits RF energy into your room, house and neighborhood, on many different frequencies.

This means that it can interfere with TV's stereos, radios, cell phones and even feedback into your electrical circuits. Even though the effect is minimal and doesn't transmit that far, you will learn from reading this book that you must have your HVAC power supply plugged into a separate outlets or preferably a different separate circuit and GFII breaker. Never plug in an NST or HVAC device on the same power strip or outlet as your expensive computer or tv's are connected to. If you have to share a strip or plug, make sure these are turned off or unplugged before your HVAC experiments begin. You can read more about this effect in the Safety Section.

Please be aware as you attempt to produce colloidal minerals that you adhere to the constraints & brewing times listed. Make sure you are using the listed batch sizes. Only when you have a good grasp on basic production methods, should you attempt to begin to experiment with other production variables. Deviation from our suggested batch sizes (32 oz or 1000ml maximum) or attempts to experiment with odd voltages and current not specifically designed for the particular colloidal mineral, might produce poor results and waste your product. Variations can also damage your colloidal power supply as well.

There are many websites that state outdated colloidal research studies that conflict about the proper way to produce colloidal products. While the tried and true method since the 1930's has used the LVDC process (an ionic - micron particle sized process) there are now many new and advanced methods will show you to produce the elusive HVAC particulate (non-ionic) Nano Colloidal solutions.

As of August 2008, the current colloidal production standard is being followed by most Canadian and US Colloidal Liquid manufacturers. This 'industry standard' method is still the old tried and proven way to produce lvdc based, ionic solutions. This method (when produced correctly) is considered safe to produce with because it uses low voltage and low dc current, making an almost 'shock-proof' experiment, even for a home user. However, the HVAC methods use 7500 through 15000 kilovolt methods and can result in severe shock hazard for the untrained colloidal producer.

By using the LVDC method and following our instructions, you'll be creating a 8-12 ppm batch of crystal clear colloidal solution that lab tests out to be about 90-95 percent IONIC colloidal .05 or better micron sized particles. You can use our methods and equipment to push a batch stronger, but there are side effects to each action passed our safety points in our methods we will teach you about. Basically, you will learn that by pushing a batch past the normal ranges, the batch begins to produce an unwanted, larger ionic particle that becomes deformed and cannot hold its charge. These causes an improperly produced batch to 'fall out of suspension' months sooner than with properly produced ionic solutions.

High Voltage methods create a 85 -95% metallic particle, called Nano particulates. These particles seem to last longer on the shelf and are said to have better bioavailable properties to fight bugs at the cellular level. It should be noted that our field results from actual HIV positive users report back that both IONIC and PARTICULATE colloidal solutions have shown an increase in their  t-cell counts and a significant decrease in their viral load lower over a three, six and nine month trial study Pride's HIV Outreach team has found. While promising, the fact's remain solid thus-far, that as of August 2008, there are NO medical studies that prove Colloidal products have every completely eradicated HIV or any other actual disease for that matter.

As with all medications, supplements and liquids, the human body absorbs and utilizes liquids, such as colloidal silver, with differing amounts of efficiency. The particle size, charge, ionic or particulate make-up, including the bodies density and cellular properties, all play a part in determining if a product is **poor** (0-6% efficiency) **stable** (6-12% efficiency) or **good** (12-20% efficiency). Delivery methods can also play a part in a products efficiency rating. Some new Nano colloidal show a larger jump in bio-efficiency, but real medical lab studies of colloidal use on real people show that a particular colloidal solution is only mildly bio-efficient. It might surprise you to know that your daily multivitamin is really only about 3-5% bio-efficient, most studies show. Some more potent liquids can only rise a bit more than those figures. Inaccurate and false websites touting Colloidal Silver as being 99% percent bio-efficient are medically and scientifically impossible.

Our results have varied, however it seems that the data that has been presented to us, shows that testing conducted in-vitro testing on staph pathogens (lab petri dishes or slides) that it was shown that both LVDC and HVAC produced Colloidal Silver killed some or all of the strains tested. These University Lab tests also proved that colloidal silver mineral product is both a natural antibiotic as well as a topical antiseptic.

Since HVAC and LVDC colloidal minerals have been effectively used for many years now, data suggests that both types of properly produced HVAC and LVDC colloidal minerals are considered safe for topical, ingestion or injected uses as a broad spectrum product. Our results have been echoed by BYU University and several medical lab studies for in vitro lab testing.

Unfortunately, most colloidal websites ask you to falsely believe that colloidal silver can effectively cure or treat many ailments, including acting as an antibiotic for human use. These dubious marketers inaccurately teach people that prescribed antibiotics are a thing of the past.

In reality, using colloidal silver to treat a serious infection is unwise and very dangerous. Colloidal therapy (even when doubling or tripling intake dosage) has been found to have about ONLY a 10-14% efficiency rating compared to taking a properly prescribed antibiotic at  50-60% efficiency rating. This means that for the organic product seeker that requires an antibiotic for a serious staph or other infection, they should be taking their prescribed medicine and should not be reliant upon only their colloidal therapy.

## Non-Scientific Control Group

One of our goals as Colloidal Science Researchers is that we'd like to see each new colloidal producer finally armed with some current and relevant manufacturing information. Even while the many production methods listed in this manual have been independently lab tested for creating an efficient, bio-available product; just as with all products we as humans place into our bodies, once they enter the body via oral means, the efficiency drops exponentially. This is true of both nano and micron styled colloidal products.

To illustrate the point, in a 2005 'real-world' quasi study conducted by Pride Scientific and several Doctor Friends over a local outbreak of staph infections. We were presented with a good pool of recently infected people requiring help or medical assistance. Some of these people Infected refused (even at our suggestion) to receive oral antibiotics, others (friends and customers) were sent to see a Medical Professional who had been researching our products and providing them at no cost to our low-income outreach as gifts.

We were able to get some real patient data from our customers that were specifically using Colloidal Therapy to treat reoccurring staph infections, while we were able to share our finding openly with medical professionals at the same time.

The group that were involved in our loose study, basically were made up of colloidal field researchers, customers and people who suffer from similar stages of strep and staph, including MRSA.

While not a controlled or blind study, we feel like our 'real world' results showed some quite promising effects of colloidal therapy. To some of the hard-core "I'm not taking prescribed antibiotics" crowd , we gave them our Multiphasic 10ppm colloidal nanosilver. At the same time the other users were prescribed strong antibiotics in the Bacterium family by a Medical Doctor. With the diagnosis being the same and almost same day infections, my Doctor buddy wanted to see how Nanosilver would affect the exact same strain of staph that his Bacterium antibiotic would affect.

Most all the colloidal users and the actual Doctor's patients freely provided lab blood tests and promised to share any discernable results to the group.

After it was all said and done, it became apparent that colloidal silver did help reduce the staph and strep infection, but at a rather slower rate than expected. Most saw their staph clear up in 14-28 days, while the bacterium seemed to clear it up in 7-14 days.

Prescribed Antibiotics won this round. But real user results proved that the colloidal therapy did assist or help the immune system fight the virus, much faster than left alone.

One side note we did learn, that those colloidal therapy users who used our '30-second-swish & swallow' method, they seemed to get better in have the time over the other colloidal users who simply drank the silver, without using the swish and then swallow method. It is therefore opined that doing the sublingual assist,  the colloidal nano particles will disperse into their bloodstream faster than by simply drinking it.

As you make colloidal therapy available to your family and friends, it is in our opinion that by using the sublingual swish method, you are increasing the bio-efficiency by about 40%.

Out of the group, the people who found the colloidal silver most effective and whose blood tests showed a decrease in the staph virus were those users that actually took time to accomplish the longer 'swish' method before swallowing.

Unfortunately, even the strongest colloidal therapy does not completely kill the virus, but it was clear that users who did the swish method saw better results in their labs and blood work, over those that did not.

The ppm strength and amount of colloidal silver (made by either ionic or particulate methods) had proven somewhat effective at fully curing the infection. The field researchers and people using the colloidal therapy path over prescribed antibiotics reported that their infections DID NOT get worse while on the colloidal products, but they couldn't completely clear it up in all cases, without finally going onto prescribed medications.

Just remember this, that if you carefully follow the production experiment instructions you'll find inside this book, you will be able to make a potentially valuable and bio-efficient alternative health supplement. Each of our methods and experiments have been tested for 'real-world' uses and both LVDC and HVAC types indicated in this manual have each been individually tested as being bioavailable and effective for easy human absorption.

The point in sharing these stories is to make you realize that most of the hype and 'new silver solution' marketing information is actually very inaccurate and false. It does not cure diseases or completely kill virus or eradicate infection. It cannot kill disease causing organisms inside the body. You cannot cure cancer, HIV/AIDS or other diseases by ingesting large amounts of colloidal products. I wished we were wrong, but actual lab tests and real pathogen kill tests show that colloidal products are not the 'major discovery' as fake web sites and advertisements suggest.

Using colloidal therapy as a supplement with other prescribed methods is a start in the right direction and nothing more. There have been thousands of studies of both medical and personal in nature, including people using IV injectable medical grade colloidal silver to treat HIV, that have shown promising, but not overwhelming cure results. If there was even a hint of a cure for cancer or HIV using colloidal products, the colloidal industry would be releasing it all over the media and pharm companies would be going nuts trying to up everything they could with colloidal methodologies. It seems that nutritional supplements seem only supplement and support the human system by making the rest of the body healthier. There are still many medical benefits to using colloidal products.

## Medical Applications

While silver, copper, zinc and other colloidal minerals all have an importance of being an actual antibacterial agent, only silver has seen the most efficiency and has been documented as a bactericide since the 1800s. Its use in purification has been known throughout the ages. Early records indicate that the Phoenicians, for example, used silver vessels to keep water, wine and vinegar pure during their long voyages. In America, early pioneers moving west put silver and copper coins in their water barrels to keep it clean of algae and fungus.

In fact, "born with a silver spoon in his mouth" is also a reference to health as well as wealth. In the early 18th century, babies who were fed with silver spoons were healthier than those fed with spoons made from other metals, and silver pacifiers found wide use in America because of their beneficial health effects. None of these millions of people over the past generations have ever turned 'blue' due to these uses of silver.

Today silver is used in many health-care products. Specifically silver sulfadiazine, which is used by every hospital in North America to prevent bacterial infections in burn victims. The silver allows the body to restore naturally the burnt tissue. It is also used worldwide under the trade name "Silvadiene."

Increasingly, wound dressings and other wound care products incorporate a layer of fabric containing tiny silver particles for prevention of secondary infections. Surgical gowns and draperies also include microscopic silver particles to prevent microbial transmission. Other medical products containing silver are catheters and stethoscope diaphragms.

In a world that is showing increasing concern about the spread of disease, silver is being increasingly tapped for its antibacterial properties. Research is ongoing on the use of silver and its compounds for therapeutic uses and on its potential use as a disinfectant in hospitals and other medical facilities.

Already, climate control system makers are using their silver laced systems on homes to airplanes to prevent the transmission of airborne bacteria that cause Legionnaires disease.

The successful preparation of nano-sized silver particles offers additional capabilities in the fight against pathogenic organisms and research programs are under way to exploit these features.

Silver is great on cuts, burns, acne, sunburn, eczema, rashes and of course, has been shown in lab Petri dishes to eradicate and smoother many disease pathogens or virus afflicting mankind today.

## Now it's time to actually save your life – Please dig into this Safety Section

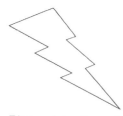 All of the methods and experiments contained in this book are accomplished through a NON-CHEMICAL process. Instead of using chemical binders and acids to make colloidal solutions, we found a better way to make a much safer, fully ingestible colloidal liquid. To make colloidal products without chemicals requires electricity, current, mineral content electrodes and a glass, of lab grade plastic batch container to ultimately design a mini electrolysis chamber.

Please take the extra time to read and understand each safety topic below, it could save your life and help you from shorting out your colloidal production equipment. Credit for this section also goes to the owners over at www.pupman.com, who are hvac enthusiasts.

### All colloidal experiments (especially the HVAC) in this guide use high voltages, and the risk of death or injury is significant. The following general guidelines are suggested

►Never adjust electrodes, wires or non-insulated clips when the power supply is turned on.

High voltage power supplies contain capacitors that may hold a charge up to 60 seconds or longer after a power supply is turned off. Always discharge the energy at the electrodes down into a batch or use the ground out method discussed later in the HVAC section before adjusting a primary circuit or electrodes. Make sure the metal cases of transformers, motors, control panels and other items associated with colloidal experiments are properly grounded.

►For High Voltage production methods (HV) make sure that you are far enough away from the corona discharge (from HVAC electrodes) so that it cannot strike you. Do not come in contact with metal objects which might be subject to a strike from the secondary or other high voltage lead set, terminal or output section of your NST HVAC colloidal power supply.

►The power supplies 120 VAC 60 Hz or 220 50 HZ (mains) low voltage primary circuits are also extremely dangerous and these voltages are especially lethal to humans. Make sure these circuits are well insulated so users cannot come in contact with the A.C. line voltage. A safety key or shut off toggle switch should be used in the low voltage circuit to prevent unauthorized use. Use adequate fusing of the primary power and/or circuit breakers to limit the maximum current to your control panel. Do NOT count on your home circuit panel to provide adequate protection!

►Never operate a plasma arc experiment or use a HV supply in an area where there is standing water, or where a significant shock hazard exists.

►Do not operate an experiment when pets or small children are present.

Lightning kills about 300 people each year in the United States, and injures an additional three to four times this number. More than one thousand people are killed each year in the U.S. due to generated electric current, and several thousand more are injured. In the case of lightning, the voltage and current are extremely high, but the duration is short. The current tends to flow on the outside of the body and may cause burns, respiratory arrest and/or cardiac arrest. Many die from lightning due to respiratory arrest rather than cardiac arrest. (The portion of the brain controlling breathing is often severely affected in a lightning strike.) Power line deaths usually involve lower voltages and currents, but the duration may be significant. Often the current flows inside the body, causing deep burns and cardiac arrest.

►While being shocked, if you are actually holding a wire, tool, etc, frequently the individual cannot let go of the power source due to involuntary muscle contraction.

The brain and heart are the most sensitive organs. The dose response for animal and human data suggest the following: for less than 10 mA hand to foot of 50-60 cycle line current, the person merely feels a "funny" sensation; for currents above 10 mA, the person freezes to the circuit and is unable to let go; For currents of 100 mA to one ampere, the likelihood of sudden death is greatest. Above one ampere, the heart is thrown into a single contraction, and internal heating becomes significant. The individual may be thrown free of the power source, but may go into respiratory and/or cardiac arrest. Six factors determine the outcome of human contact with electrical current: voltage, amperage, resistance, frequency, duration and pathway. I will discuss each individually.

**Voltage** Low voltages generally do not cause electrical shocks that are severe enough to cause any injury unless the external resistance is low (so don't fire up your experiment on wet floor areas). As the voltage is increased, more and more current passes through the body, possibly causing damage to the brain, heart, or causing involuntary muscle contractions. Perhaps 100-250 volts A. C. is the most lethal voltage, because it is high enough to cause significant current flow through the body, and may cause muscles to contract tightly, rendering the victim incapable of letting go. Lower voltages often are insufficient to cause enough current flow, and higher voltages may cause the victim to be thrown clear of the hazard due to the particularly fierce involuntary muscle contractions. Arcing may occur with high voltages, however. Naturally, burns become more severe as the voltage is increased.

**Amperage IS Current** Greater amperage means greater damage, especially due to heating within tissues. As little as 10 microamps of current passing directly through the heart can cause ventricular fibrillation (heart muscle fibers beat out of sync, so no blood is pumped) and cardiac arrest. Because of the air filled lungs, much of the current passing through the chest may potentially pass through the heart. The spinal cord may also be affected, altering respiration control. 100 ma to 1 amp is sufficient to induce respiratory arrest and/or cardiac arrest. (Most LVDC Colloidal Power comes preset to around 33.1 vdc max at under 10 ma.) Thermal heating of tissues increases with the square of the current (I2R), so high current levels can cause severe burns, which may be internal.

**Resistance** A heavily callused dry palm may have a resistance of 1 megohm. A thin, wet palm may register 100 ohms of resistance (wet hands are bad). Resistance is lower in children. Different body tissues exhibit a range of resistances. Nerves, arteries and muscle are low in resistance. Bone, fat and tendon are relatively high in resistance. Across the chest of an average adult, the resistance is about 70-100 ohms. Thermal burns due to I2R losses in the body can be significant, resulting in the loss of life or limb long after the initial incident. A limb diameter determines the approximate "cross section" which the current will flow through, (for moderate voltages and low frequencies). As a result, a current passing through the arm generates more temperature rise and causes more thermal damage than when passing through the abdomen.

**Frequency** The "skin effect" also applies to a human conductor, and as the frequency gets above about 500 kHz or so, little energy passes through the internal organs. Most colloidal outputs operate between 150 hz through 15 khz range, where we operate most LVDC and HVAC power outputs. At a given voltage, 50-60 hz A.C. current has a much greater ability to cause ventricular fibrillation than D.C. current. In addition, at 50-60 Hz, involuntary muscle contractions may be so severe that the individual cannot let go of the power source. The higher frequencies we use for colloidal generation are less able to cause these involuntary contractions.

**Pathway** Obviously, the longer the duration, the more severe the internal heating of tissues. Duration is particularly a problem when working with 110-240 volts A.C., which can render the individual incapable of letting go. If the current passes through the brain or heart, the likelihood of a lethal dose increases significantly. For example, hand to hand current flow carries a 60% mortality, whereas hand to foot current flow results in 20% overall mortality. Be aware that foot to foot conduction can also occur, if a high voltage lead is inadvertently stepped on or if grounding is inadequate.

**Electrical Precautions** Obviously, the A.C. line voltage, the high voltage transformer and the high voltage R.F. generated by a HVAC NST colloidal arc experiment are each potentially lethal in their own unique way, one must always respect this extreme danger and use high voltage shielding, contactors, safety interlocks, careful R.F. and A.C. grounding, and safe operating procedures when working with such power supplies..

A safety key to prevent inexperienced operators from energizing a HVAC supply is essential. High voltage capacitors can also retain lethal energies (especially in the "equidrive" configuration) and should always be grounded before adjusting a primary. Whenever possible, have a buddy around to assist you.

Place one hand in your pocket when near electrical components so the current won't pass through your chest, and use the back of your hand to touch any electrical components so you can let go if it happens to bite you. Remember that most deaths are caused by regular 110-120 VAC house power, never perform experiments when overtired or under the influence of mind altering drugs.

**Electrical Dangers** Exposed wiring on transformers. Most NST HVAC transformers have exposed high voltage lugs or alligator clips/leads.

A 15000 volt transformer has a turn ratio of 125:1 (assuming 120 volts in). If you haven't disconnected your input power from the source (unplugged your variac), you may be in for a surprise. A variac that is putting out two volts will give you a 250 volt shock if you touch the high voltage outputs of the neon sign transformer. Once I shocked myself with one end (7500 volts) of a 60 mA. neon sign transformer. I just brushed against an exposed end, so I wasn't gripping anything. It was quite painful, much more so than touching a sparkplug wire. I felt the path of the current follow my arm, and go down my leg. Keep one hand in your pocket when working near or with charged items. (Capacitors, secondary coils, etc.)

**Charged capacitors** Older power supplies and NST's will almost always have a residual charge remaining on the capacitor when the system is turned off. Capacitors can "regain" charge from dielectric "memory". The charge remains after the capacitor has been discharged. Later the molecules return to their original states and the charge that they "captured" ends up on the plates of the capacitor. This charge is then available to shock you.

**Other sources of danger** If you isolate your own body well away from the floor and any other potentially conductive objects in the vicinity, such as sitting or standing on an elevated insulated platform (I would NOT consider a plastic milk crate adequate) then you will probably survive if 60 Hz is introduced into the streamer you are in contact with by the mechanism described above. However, in setting up this insulated platform you must consider the path that may be taken from streamers that will re-emerge from your body and head off looking for other targets, which could result in direct contact with earth ground again. The 60 cycle side of things is where electrocution can happen. Keep well away from any 60 cycle leads, use grounds and cages as appropriate. Bear in mind that if a radio frequency arc starts from a place which also has 60 cycles on it (one side of a primary circuit, for example) there is the possibility of high-current 60 cycle conduction along the ionized path. That could be deadly, so just remember to ISOLATE yourself from HOT or LIVE wires, clips, electrodes and parts at all times and you will hopefully never get a shock. Now, with that being said, all the NST HVAC units we sell, include a full ground fault auto limiting circuit. When it sees a short, such as a shock into human flesh, the unit automatically powers back to a few thousand volts at very little amperage. This doesn't mean the circuit will stop you from being electrocuted, but it may reduce any damage to that of a small shock or burn, without causing any bodily harm.

**Burns** HVAC powered clips and electrodes while under power can cause burns, especially due to RF discharges from the secondary outputs or the arc. Stay out of the immediate vicinity of a HVAC arc experiment, don't touch the lead sets, glass or plastic beakers or place a TDS meter into an ONGOING HVAC batch or you'll zap it forever. Remember, if you do get zapped by a NST or HVAC system, the heating effects may be mostly internal, causing lasting damage! Also remember that spark gaps and electrode tips get hot and are a potential source of burns.

**Induction Field Effect**  HVAC arc experiments operate in a pulsed mode, and strong electric and magnetic fields are locally produced. In addition, significant amounts of RF may be produced if the grounding is poor, or before spark breakout. This can result in induced currents in other conductors, like test equipment, nearby computers and electronics, and metal structures in the facility. The end result is generally bad. Turn off computers and sensitive test equipment, and move it away from the vicinity of your coils.

Do not plug in your NST HV power supply into the same circuit as your TV, stereo or computer. If you foolishly choose to use your house electrical ground as your RF ground, you are asking for trouble. Currents may be induced anywhere in the building, and voltage standing waves along the wiring may destroy electronics far from the HVAC experiment location.

Construct a dedicated RF ground, and make sure it is properly connected before firing any HVAC unit above substantial size. Most grounded NST and HVAC power supplies seem to work ok on good GFII circuits.

**Static charges**  During the operation of the HVAC experiment, the batch waters usually ground out some of the static discharge caused by the Underwater Plasma Arc methods we teach, however, significant static charges can build up on the lead sets and alligator clips to the electrodes. If you need to move the secondary (say you are adjusting the electrode for a better continuous arc), you may get a nasty zap right across your chest when you pick it up with both hands.

It is best NOT to touch an ongoing experiment, but sometimes it is necessary to adjust the electrode spark gap to maintain the plasma arc. Use a fully insulated tool such as a plastic tube or rod to hit or nudge your leads, alligator clips or the electrode wire slightly to get it arcing continuously once again. Never use your hands or fingers to adjust an ongoing experiment. This includes NOT TOUCHING red/b lack or white leads).
Before you touch the secondary, wipe it lightly with a grounded wire or use plastic or wooden pliers and tools. You can sometimes hear the crackling as you do so. Besides the shock hazard, there is the physical hazard caused by the shock. You will likely drop the secondary or jump onto something that isn't soft.

**Hazards of High Voltage Circuits**  Strikes to house electrical ground -- also goes to power(?) A HVAC system must be connected to a ground that is separate from the house ground or water pipes for the best practice. Connecting your HVAC systems to either of these grounds is a recipe for disaster. Notice that your stereo, computer, VCR, etc., have three prong plugs. Also, note where your telephone box is grounded. It is likely grounded to the water pipes.

Electric fields inducing currents and killing sensitive meters. Oddly enough sensitive meters and measuring equipment are just that -- sensitive. Solid state instruments are much more susceptible to damage from being near HVAC operational experiments than are vacuum tube items. Consider purchasing a cheap volt-ohmeter (VOM) with an analog meter movement. If will survive in places many digital units will not..

**Good electrical practice**  Place your HVAC power supply system in a location that will prevent the strikes from hitting electrical outlets, people, animals, and sensitive electrical equipment. Turn off and unplug computers in your house.

**Ozone, NOx, and Vapors**  A sparking (open air) plasma arc produces ozone and nitrogen-oxygen compounds, but underwater arc experiments don't have access to the air needing to metabolize these substances in any great amount. It is important not to cover a plasma underwater arc. It is also import to let your batch breathe and let what little vapors created naturally bleed off into the air. Keep an open window in your home lab to make sure you don't build up ozone.

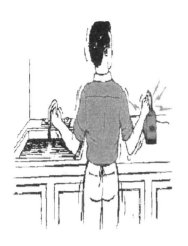

<u>Ultraviolet Light and X-ray Production</u>  Ultraviolet light may be produced by the spark gap during operation of a arc experiment. The human eye has no pain sensors within it, so the bioeffects are felt later, when it is too late. Ever look at the sun for a while, or watch a welder at work? The light produced in a spark gap (even underwater) is essentially identical to that produced by an arc welder, containing substantial amounts of hard ultraviolet light. Don't sit and stare at it, even though it is amazing to behold! As any professional arc welder will tell you "Don't Look At The Arc!" The visible light is extremely bright, and the ultraviolet light will damage your eyes, and can cause skin cancer. The arc is so bright that you couldn't make out any detail anyway, so why bother? If you must study your spark gap, use welder's glasses. Generally, it is not too difficult to rig up a piece of plastic, cardboard, etc. that will shield yourself and others. Remember that an underwater arc is about 500 times less bright than the same arc burning O2 out in the open air.

<u>Radio Frequency Interference</u>  Underwater arc experiment are continually grounding out into the water base, however, they do still produce a fair amount of RF, especially if operated with a large top capacitance, before spark breakout. Significant quantities of RF can also be produced if the RF grounding is inadequate. This can cause interference with TV's, radios, and other electronics. If you note interference, try to improve your ground first, since that is likely where your problem is. In addition, every HVAC power supply should be wired with a power line conditioner in series with the primary circuit. These are relatively inexpensive and are very effective in keeping RF out of the house wiring. NEVER PLUG IN AN NST or HVAC power supply into the same outlet as a Computer, stereo, radio, TV that is actually turned on. In fact, it is BEST to pull the plug of these electrical sensitive devices while running an HVAC batch.

Most of the Colloidal Experiments we will discuss in this book are 30 mA and under. The Author took a 15,000 volt 60 mA charge up his left arm and through his chest and down his right arm to ground.
The effect was a very sore (like I just picked up a car off a crushed kid) 'like' feeling that lasted for a day. No other physical side effects were reported. But this 'stupidity' of brushing my arm against a beaker of HVAC Nanosilver being made, while simultaneously holding onto a separate metal, plugged in lab tester, could have stopped my heart.
Never become part of the circuit.

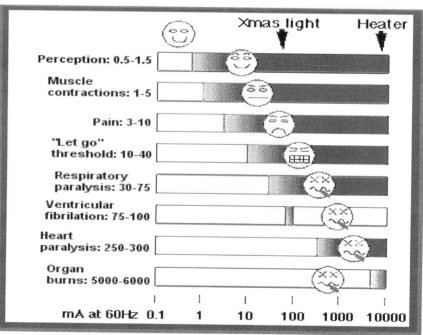

**If you are unsure of your set up and surroundings PLEASE email Marc or call Pride Scientific to discuss your setup lab concerns before attempting to manufacture your very first batch.**

# Colloidal Regulations & Production Help

As already mentioned in the forward section, the manufacturing, brewing, distilling and selling of colloidal minerals in the United States is regulated by the Food & Drug Administration, Environmental Protection Agency and the Dietary Supplement Health and Education Act. In Canada, colloidal products are regulated as well. Also new 10ppm strength requirements have been imposed in New Zealand and now Australia.

We suggest that you seriously look into your local, state and federal laws too see if you can legally manufacturer, posses or market your finished products.

In trying to help keep you legal, here is how we interrupt the DSHEA data.

"Nutritional Support" Statements"  DSHEA allows dietary supplements to bear **"statements of support"** that: (a) claim a benefit related to classical nutrient deficiency disease; (b) describe how ingredients affect the structure or function of the human body; (c) characterize the documented mechanism by which the ingredients act to maintain structure or function; and (d) describe general well-being from consumption of the ingredients. The statement "calcium builds strong bones and teeth" is said to be a classic example of an allowable structure/function statement for a food. What constitutes an allowable statement for a supplement has not been established either by law or by regulation.

To be legal under DSHEA, a "nutritional support" statement must not be a "drug" claim. In other words, it should not suggest that the product or its ingredient is intended for prevention or treatment of disease. However, the marketplace has been flooded by statements related to organs (such as "supports the eyes" or "supports the cardiovascular system") that are really drug claims.

Actually, few statements about the biochemical or physiologic properties of nutrients have practical value for consumers. By definition, every essential nutrient is important to proper body function. Simple statements about nutrient function are more likely to be misleading than helpful. A statement such as "vitamin A is essential to good eye function" could suggest: (a) people need to take special steps to be sure they get enough, (b) extra vitamin A may enhance eyesight, and (c) common eye problems may be caused vitamin A deficiency or remedies by taking supplements.

To be completely truthful, a "nutritional support" statement about vitamin A would have to counter all three misconceptions and indicate that people eating sensibly don't need to worry about whether their vitamin A intake is adequate. In other words, truthful statements about nutrient supplements would have to indicate who doesn't need them. No vitamin manufacturer has ever done this or ever will. Since herbs are not nutrients, the concept of "nutritional support" statements for herbs is absurd. Under DSHEA, manufacturers who make statements of "nutritional support" must have substantiation that such statements are truthful and not misleading. The law also requires that the Secretary of Health and Human Services be notified no later than 30 days after the first marketing of a supplement for which the statement is being made. The law does not define substantiation.

Historically, the FDA has considered literature used directly in connection with the sale of a product to be "labeling" for the product. DSHEA exempts publications from "labeling" if they: (a) are not false or misleading, (b) do not promote a particular manufacturer or brand, (c) present a "balanced" view of pertinent scientific information, and (d) are physically separated from the items discussed. However, since most "dietary supplements" are useless, irrationally formulated, and/or overpriced, the supplement industry has little reason to provide literature that is not misleading. In addition, the FDA does not have the resources to police the huge numbers of "support" statements to ensure that they are appropriately "balanced."  To be legal, you should be producing products labels and/or information for sale that states: 'Dietary Supplement' as well as with the Ingredients, bottle size in ounces or milliliters and dosing information if you have room.

## New Rules in 1998-2008

To help you produce and label your items correctly, there are new rules for statements about the effect of dietary supplement products on body structure and function. These rules included:

Disease claims are not permitted. Disease is defined as "any deviation from, impairment of, or interruption of the normal structure or function of any part, organ, or system (or combination thereof of the body that is manifested by a characteristic set of one or more signs or symptoms."

"Signs or symptoms" include laboratory or clinical assessments that are characteristic of a disease, such as an elevated cholesterol fraction, uric acid, or blood sugar, and characteristic signs of disease, such as elevated blood pressure. A claim that a product helps protect against a disease (e.g., "reduces the stiffness of arthritis") is a disease claim. Some manufacturers state "supports bones and joints" to get around the requirement statements.

A product name that implies an effect on a disease, e.g. "Hepatocure" would constitute a disease claim, but names such as "Cardiohealth" or "Heart Tabs" would not. Suggestions that a product helps fight a specific disease or type of disease by stimulating the body's defenses would be disease claims, but "general claims such as "supports the immune system" would not [12].

On January 6, 2000, after receiving more than 100,000 protest messages from the supplement industry and its allies, the FDA published a revised final rule on health claims for dietary supplements [13,14]. DSHEA permits claims that products affect the structure or function of the body, provided the manufacturer has substantiating documents on file. Without prior FDA review, products may not bear a claim that they can prevent, treat, cure, mitigate or diagnose disease. The final rule still prohibits express disease claims (such as "prevents osteoporosis"), and implied disease claims ("prevents bone fragility in postmenopausal women"), including claims made through a product's name ("CircuCure") or through pictures or symbols.

The rule permits health-maintenance claims ("maintains a healthy circulatory system"); other non-disease claims ("for muscle enhancement," "helps you relax,"); and claims for common, minor symptoms associated with pregnancy, menopause, or other life stages (e.g., "for common symptoms of PMS," "for hot flashes"). However, osteoporosis and other serious conditions associated with aging, menopause or adolescence will still be treated as diseases.

## FDA Requirements

If you intend to market and sell your products, somewhere on your catalogs and website should be the basic following FDA disclaimer.

*"The products and the claims made about specific products on or through this site have not been evaluated by the United States Food and Drug Administration and are not approved to diagnose, treat, cure or prevent disease. The information provided on this site is for informational purposes only and is not intended as a substitute for advice from your physician or other health care professional or any information contained on or in any product label or packaging. You should not use the information on this site for diagnosis or treatment of any health problem or for prescription of any medication or other treatment.*

*You should consult with a healthcare professional before starting any diet, exercise or supplementation program, before taking any medication, or if you have or suspect you might have a health problem. Please view our full Terms of Use and Disclaimer for more information and the terms and conditions governing your use of this site."*

## Colloidal Therapy and Results

The Colloidal Therapy phrase basically means the ingestion or topical use of colloidal silver, copper, gold, zinc or copper, or any combination thereof. When ingested, certain minerals can make your natural levels change as well. For instance, using too much copper can disturbed your natural zinc and other levels, so please start out any colloidal therapy by using small amounts. You should never ingest more than two ounces of silver, zinc or gold in a 24 hour period. You should never ingest more than a tablespoon of liquid copper per 24 hour period.

Below is a list of what people who are involved with colloidal therapies SAY they are using it for. Remember, this is what customers and field researchers report using it for; we are making no claims as to the accuracy of colloidal use on any of the ailments listed below.

### Ionic or Nano-Particulate Colloidal Silver as an alternative to Antibiotics:

Food Preservation, Household Disinfectant, Acne, Arthritis (see gold), Athlete's Foot, Blastocystis Hominous, Burns, Cancer, Chronic Diarrhea, Cold & Flu (see zinc also), Hayfever Allergies, Cuts, Wounds and Sores, Ear Infections, Emphysema, Eye Infections, Fungal Infections & Candida, Giardia Lamblia, Head lice (see RID instead), Herpes, Hepatitis B and C, High Blood Pressure (see gold also), Lyme Disease, Osteomyelitis, Psoriasis (see zinc & copper), Ringworm, Shingles, Sinus Infections, Strep & Staph Infections, Skin Infections, Scars, Surgery, Throat Infections, Ulcerative Colitis, Urinary Tract Infections, Warts, Yeast Infections.

### Ionic or Nano Particulate Zinc (or combo silver-zinc)

Cold & Flu use, skin conditions, Psoriasis, Eczema.

### Ionic or Nano Particulate Copper

Topical use is recommended; used as additives for skin creams, anti-wrinkle creams and graying hair in shampoos.

### Nano Particulate Gold

Arthritis, joint pain, meditation, neural pathways, past life regression, massage oils, etc.

SIlverGen has a nice list of other uses they have compiled for Colloidal Silver, here is their abbreviated list:

Add to suspected drinking water when traveling or camping. Silver-sprayed burns heal rapidly without scarring. Safely sterilize anything from toothbrushes to surgical instruments. Use topically on cuts, wounds, abrasions, rashes, sunburn, insect bites, razor nicks and bandages. Spray on garbage to prevent decay odors. Mist kitchen sponges, towels, cutting boards to eliminate E. Coli and salmonella bacteria to prevent food poisoning and gastrointestinal inflammation. Add when canning, preserving or bottling.

Use like peroxide on zits and acne. Add to juices and milk to prevent spoiling, fermenting, deteriorating, clabbering or curdling. Spray in shoes and between toes to stop most skin itch, athlete's foot and fungi. Diminish dandruff, psoriasis, skin rashes, etc. Add to bath water, gargle, douches, colon irrigation, nasal spray and dental water-pic solutions.

Cuts downtime dramatically from colds, flu, pneumonia, staph, strep, respiratory infections and rhino viruses. Skin itch, eye irritation or infection (dilute a small amount with an equal amount of distilled water for eye use) and ear infections (warm slightly first), some moles and warts vanish (put on band aid pad and wear on wart overnight each night until gone).

Use with Q-tips on fingernail, toenail, and ear fungi. Can impede tooth decay and bad breath. Unlike pharmaceutical antibiotics, Colloidal Silver never permits strain-resistant pathogens to evolve. Toothaches, mouth sores, bacterial irritations are diminished. Soak dentures.
Spray refrigerator, freezer and food storage bin interiors.

Mix in postage stamp, envelope, and tape moistening wells, paint and paste pots to prevent bacterial growth, odors, spoiling or souring. Add to water-based paints, wallpaper paste, dishwater, cleaning and mopping solutions, etc. Spray pet bedding and let dry. Spray on top of contents of opened jam, jelly, and condiment containers and inside lids before replacing.
Mix a little in pet water, birdbaths, cut flower vases.

Add to swamp cooler water. Spray air conditioner filters after cleaning. Swab air ducts and vents to prevent breeding sites for germs. Use routinely in laundry final rinse water and always before packing away seasonal clothes.
Damp clothes or towels and washcloths will not sour or mildew. Eliminate unwanted microorganisms in planter soils and hydroponics systems. Spray plant foliage to stop fungi, molds, rot, and most plant diseases.
Silver is an excellent plant-growth stimulator. Treat pools, fountains, humidifiers, Jacuzzis, hot tubs, baths, and dishwashers, re-circulating cooling tower water, gymnasium foot dips, and bath and shower mats. Spray inside shoes, watch bands and gloves and under fingernails periodically.

Treat shower stalls, tubs, fonts, animal watering troughs, shavers to avoid trading germs. Rinse fruit and vegetables before storing or using. Put in cooking water. Add to human and animal shampoos and they become disinfectants.

Prevent carpets, drapes and wallpaper from mildewing. Wipe telephone mouthpieces, pipe stems, headphones, hearing aids, eyeglass frames, hairbrushes, combs, loofas. Excellent for diapers and diaper rash. Spray toilet seats, bowls, tile floors, sinks, urinals, door knobs. Kills persistent odors. Rinse invalid's pillowcases, sheets, towels and bedclothes. There are literally thousands of other essential uses for this odorless, nearly tasteless and colorless, totally benign, powerful, non-toxic disinfectant and healing agent. You'll find that a spray or misting bottle of Colloidal Silver solution may be the most useful health enhancement tool in your environment.

## So, what about dosage?

Some people, when first ingesting Colloidal Silver, have the experience that is called the **Herxheimer** effect.

This experience is a result of the silver very efficiently killing off **too many** pathogens too fast for the body to dispose of through the normal eliminative organs. This forces the body to utilize the secondary eliminative organs: the lungs, sinuses and skin. Sometimes this causes a few days of flu-like symptoms. This is normal when starting an effective colloidal therapy regime. Everyone has 'GOOD FLORA' in their system, when you take too much colloidal silver, it not only kills off the bad bacteria, but the good bacteria called 'flora' as well.

Sometimes a new Colloidal Silver user who ingests Colloidal Silver for the first time will experience what feels like a cold or the flu (or diarrhea) symptoms. This can be stopped by cutting back on the dosage (or completely abstaining for a day or so), or prevented by starting with a small dose (1/4 to 1 teaspoon twice a day) and gradually increasing the dosage. We suggest that new users and even those daily users of colloidal silver, take a PROBIOTIC capsule daily or eat one cup of YOGURT daily to keep the 'good flora' in your system from being killed off by the potent colloidal silver.

## Ingesting Colloidal Silver (similar dosage requirement for zinc, copper and gold as well)

Taken orally, the silver solution is absorbed from the mouth into the bloodstream, and then transported quickly to the body cells. Swishing the solution under the tongue for **30 seconds** before swallowing results in faster absorption of any colloidal product. In three to four days the silver may accumulate in the tissues sufficiently for benefits to begin. Colloidal silver is eliminated by the kidneys, lymph system and bowel after several days or even weeks.

## Chronic or Serious Conditions

1-2 TABLESPOONS of 5 to 10ppm in morning and later right before bed at night. Most IONIC 5 ppm. Colloidal silver equals about 25 micrograms (mcg.) of silver. 1 - 4 tablespoons per day (25 - 100 mcg.) is generally considered to be a "nutritional amount" and is reported to be safe to use for extended periods of time.

Amounts higher than this are generally considered "therapeutic amounts" and should only be used periodically. In cases of illness, natural health practitioners have often recommended taking double or triple the "nutritional amount" for 30 to 45 days, then dropping down to a smaller maintenance dose.

Amounts from 1 to 6 ounces per day have reportedly been used in acute conditions. If your body is extremely ill or toxic, do not be in a hurry to clear up everything at once. If pathogens are killed off too quickly, the body's five eliminatory channels (liver, kidneys, skin, lungs and bowel) may be temporarily overloaded, causing flu-like conditions, headache, extreme fatigue, dizziness, nausea or aching muscles.

### Actual HIV Case note and Lab blood test results:

Hello, my name is **** *****  and I live in Portland, Oregon and have advanced HIV. I have tried MesoSilver and *ASAP silver and quite frankly could NOT AFFORD them anymore. I was seeing expense without results! *Asap silver is actually Nutronix 'New Silver Solution' a supposedly patented process who was recently investigated by the FDA.

My counts were down and my viral load was up and I was just about a month out from going onto the destructive HIV medications, but as a last resort I found PRIDELABS HIV Outreach on the net. I told them my plight and was given two new (500ml) bottles of MultiPhasic Colloidal Silver to try. Here are my actual results based upon my lab blood tests.

 I could not believe the results from this NEW TYPE of Colloidal Silver that uses nano particles to help fight viruses like mine. This wiped out almost half of my HIV in just two and a half months and my tests PROVE IT!

Viral Load September 20, 2007 came in at 42,300 copies/ml and I started on just the MultiPhasic Colloidal Therapy and on 12/13/07 I got tested again by the same lab and after almost two and a half months on Colloidal Therapy, my viral load is down to  27,900 copies/ml. A consistent 34% drop in the amount of HIV in my system! I'm not on any other medications except for MultiPhasic Colloidal Silver. My February 2008 results also showed an improvement and my viral load was down at around 22,500 copies/ml.

## Technical Terms & Data Information

### Ionic Colloidal Particle

Any electro generated particle (Usually under .05 micron range) that is produced inside a distilled or de-ionized water base by placing precise and controlled LVDC voltage onto two Silver, Gold, Copper, Zinc, Platinum electrodes, suspended in the liquid base.

### Particulate Colloidal Particle (referred to by the industry as NanoColloidal Particles)

Any electro generated particle (Usually in the nano particulate range of 3-100nm particle) that is produced inside a distilled water base by placing HVAC onto two Silver, Gold, Copper, Zinc, Platinum electrodes, suspended in the liquid base.

### Colloidal Silver

A Colloidal Liquid, with an actual amount of small silver particles, unseen by the human eye, that is said to be beneficial to aiding the human, animal and plant immune systems. Colloidal Silver should be CRYSTAL CLEAR in all forms to be safe.

### Colloidal Gold

A Colloidal Liquid, with an actual amount of small 24k gold particles, unseen by the human eye, that is said to be beneficial to aiding the human and animal with joint pain, arthritis, swelling, and even has a mild mood elevating by-product. Colloidal Gold is usually light pink or reddish or can be clear. Dark colors like ruby red or violet indicate a wasteful product containing too large of particles to be effectively introduced into the body and instead gets wasted out by bodily function. With gold almost at $900 per ounce, this is silly to push NANOGOLD to such high ppm's when low 3-5ppm works great for Arthritis, PMS and other joint, back pain. Larger particles of any mineral are undesirable, because they can store in your fatty tissues and cause toxicity and heavy metal poisoning.

### Constant Current

The proper electronic term is Current Regulated. Any regulated lab grade or even some non-lab grade power supply carry some amount of current regulation. Regulation helps steady the colloidal batch throughout it's changing current draw and voltage needs. 9 volt battery designs do not contain any regulation and are therefore NOT CONSTANT CURRENT power supplies. *This does not apply to HVAC systems.

**LVDC** stands for Low Voltage Direct Current, usually 27 to 36 VDC and anywhere from 5ma to 3 amps constant current.

**HVDC** stands for High Voltage Direct Current, usually 100 - 300 VDC and anywhere from 10ma to 20 amps.

**HVAC** stands for High Voltage AC, usually around 2500 VAC to 15,000 VAC and about 20 to 50 ma.

**NST** This is a type of High Voltage Power supply minimally required to produce Nano-Particulate colloidal minerals. 4500 Volts is about the lowest you would want to produce with. 9k or 15 k @ 15-30 ma works best.

## SLP EFFECT: Site Location Probabilities Effect

The SLP effect somewhat hampers a consistent Colloidal Production, even in clean lab environments. Some of the SLP's that can affect your regular colloidal production are:

**Your location, temperature in the room, temperature of your liquid base waters, altitude, barometric pressure, humidity, dew-point, voltage & current, purity of liquid water base and finally the purity of your minerals and lab production accessories.**

While experimenting on making your own colloidal batch, you will notice very soon that the SLP effect will make your batches progress and change differently (slightly) every day. Even in a clean lab, with climate controlled conditions, we see the SLP affect a batch differently each brewing session. A side note about producing in the desert states, it does seem that producing batches on cold, humid days makes quicker, more potent batches, while on hot, dry days, make a slower batch. The only way for labs NOT be hampered by these SLP effects seem to be by producing colloidal minerals inside a sealed vacuum chamber or argon gas chamber to simulate a vacuum, oxygen free area. In reality, the SLP effect is very manageable for daily production sessions and the effect is not as bad as one would think, once the colloidal producer gets a good baseline, production system operating..

**Silver IONS (Ag+)** – An ion of silver is formed when a single electron is removed from a silver atom causing the ion to have a positive charge. An ion that has a positive charge is attracted to the cathode and is referred to as a cathode ion. Silver ions are water-soluble and exist only in the presence of water or other solvent . Silver ions diffuse through a solution due to the mutual repulsion they have for each other caused by their ionic charge . Silver ions exist as individual entities in solution and do not cluster together to form particles like atoms. A silver ion is a different form of matter than an atom of silver and has entirely different physical properties. While an ion possesses ionic charge owing to the missing electron, it is not considered an atom of silver with a charge. Ionic charge is caused by the missing electron and is different from particle charge that is caused by adsorption of ions on the surface of the particle. If the water containing silver ions is evaporated, the ions are forced to combine with anions present in the solution and will thus become a silver compound when the water is removed. The silver compound(s) produced is determined by the anions present in the solution before the water is removed. Silver ions do contribute to the electrical conductivity of solutions that contain them. Adding silver ions to the solution does increase the conductivity. Silver ions are soluble in water and do combine readily to form compounds.

**Silver Particles** – Particles are clusters of silver atoms . The size of the particles found in a colloid can range in size from 1 nanometer (nm) to 1000 nm. The size of the particles typically found in silver colloids is under 1000 nm. The atoms in a silver particle remain held together by van der Waals' force of attraction that causes like (identical) atoms to be attracted to each other. A particle 1 nm in diameter consists of 31 silver atoms, a particle 10 nm in diameter consists of about 31000 atoms and a particle 20 nm in diameter consists of about 250,000 atoms. Silver metallic (HV methods) particles do not heavily contribute to the electrical conductivity of solutions that contain them. So PPM and TDS meters have some trouble with them, where-as on an Ionic, LVDC Batch, the meters are fairly accurate. Adding silver particles to the solution does not wildly increase the conductivity. There is varying research in the IONIC to PARTICULATE ratio arena, mostly different information from one manufacturer to another about which is best. Here is what we know about our systems. DIGIPRO LVDC systems create a mostly IONIC colloidal product. When producing one 32 oz batch of 10 ppm crystal clear silver, our outside lab testing reported that the PS05, PS10, PS30, PS50, PS75, PS120, PS400 and DUALPORT models all create about an **90-95% IONIC** silver particle and the uniform particle sizes were at or near .05 microns respectively. The remaining 5-10% was actual metallic, silver particulate in the high nano range of 100 nm uniform size respectively. This is an important number when LVDC generator shopping as most manufacturers don't know their units output ratios or have never had a separate lab test done to prove their designs. Research in colloidal products absorption and bioavailability effectiveness has a direct correlation to how small the actual silver charged particle is. The smaller the particle, the easier to absorb and affect the body's pathogens at the cellular level.

DIGIPRO NST HVAC or PLASMA ARC systems such as the NST, PS15, PS100, PS200 and PS1000 all produce a **99% nano particulate** silver, copper, zinc and gold. Outside testing reveals that a 10 ppm batch of Nano Silver (32 oz batch) tests out to be about 3 to 15 nanometers in size. There are occasionally larger clusters and chunks about 100 nm when dealing with arc processes for gold production.

**Electrical Conductivity** - The measurement of electrical conductivity is generally referred to as just conductivity. Conductivity is the reciprocal of the receptivity of a material. When a fluid is involved, the

Electrolytic conductivity is given by the ratio of current density to the electric field strength. The conductance of a sample of pure water depends on how the measurement was made. Things that affect conductance include how big a sample is being measured, how far apart the electrodes are, etc. Conductance is defined as the reciprocal of the resistance in ohms, measured between the opposing faces of a 1 cm cube of liquid at a specific temperature. The unit of conductance is called Siemens (S) which was formerly named the mho (ohm spelled backward). Because a measurement gives the conductance, methods have been devised to convert the measured value to the conductivity, so that results can be compared from different experiments. The unit of conductivity is Siemens/m or in scaled form Siemens/cm. An approximation of the concentration of ionic silver in solution (ppm) may be determined from the conductivity.

## PARTICULATE and IONIC AMOUNTS in actual Colloidal Products (based on lab tests)

If you produce 10ppm of Ionic (LVDC) produced silver, copper or zinc, the following basic formula is pretty accurate:

10 PPM of measure Ionic Colloidal Silver contains **about** 10,000 mcg per 1000 ml batch.
So, a 16 oz bottle is about 500ml and half of the quart batch, so you can assume that if your batch measures in at 10ppm, a 16 ounce final batch will have 5,000 mcg per bottle or 64 tablespoons of 78 mcg's each tablespoon. This is well below the EPA's toxicity alert warning levels.

Normal intake by and adult should be a full tablespoon two times daily. Children under 12 should be half that. If severe sore throat or viral stuff is going on, I have my family take about 1 oz in the morning and another full ounce later that night. Taking it during the onset of colds and flu seem to lesson the symptoms and speed up overall recovery time by about 30-40%. SWISH and HOLD the colloidal liquid inside the mouth for a full 30 seconds before swallowing for best effect.

**Colloidal Gold** sinters off at a slower rate using the HVAC PAUM, as gold is the most conductive and yet most permeable substance on earth. In other words, it sticks together no matter what!

The actual mcg's of CG products are based on preliminary data only, actual independent lab tests should be done by your own lab if making any products for commercial consumption. When properly produced, 5ppm of CG in quart batch container 1,500 mcg's were found, so a 16 ounce bottle would have 750 mcg's of particle colloidal gold in each bottle.

## The ideal LVDC or HVAC Colloidal Silver Solution

Despite which method you use, we want to see a **CLEAR COLLOIDAL SILVER**, with a total measurement (LVDC methods) of around 5ppm up to maybe 10ppm maximum. For MHVDC and HVAC systems, you will be able to make anywhere from 5 to 10 ppm.

Believe it or not, the HIGHER the ppm level does not make a particular batch 'stronger' it only makes the batch have more larger, unusable particle that can be wasted away by the body. What we don't want to see is a dark golden or outrageously high ppm silver. Some colloidal silver, when it has progressed too far, will turn yellow or golden brown or even gray. Please don't ingest this, but don't destroy the batch either as you can still use it for topical creams or plant fuel.

The higher the actual ppm of a given batch gets, compounded with its changing color, usually indicates that the SILVER PARTICLES have begun to double and triple in size. The particles are now becoming conglomerated into bigger silver clusters. When the particle clusters get big enough, the clusters begin to reflect light and are actually big enough that the human eye can now perceive them as colored wavelengths.

These conglomerated particles have grown so large that they reflect light in the yellow or gray color spectrum. Keep your batches in the clear range so that you will always know your particle is the smallest size for easier absorption. Clear colloidal silver has only a slight electrical or metallic after taste, this is normal and if you desire less taste, make a lighter 5ppm batch, want more silver, make a 15 ppm silver batch.

It is possible to make pure, LVDC generated clear colloidal silver up to the 20 ppm, but it depends on your SLP effect and lab setup. This higher 20 ppm result (while maintaining the clear color) can be accomplished only if you start with good generation equipment and really pure distilled water.

You really want to maximize the ppm strength without causing the color shift. This is the PERIOD right before the saturation point, or when the batch starts to take the color turn. This period can vary slightly from day to day and from batch to batch. Something that producers need to do more of is to cover batches when they complete them and let stand for 12 to 24 hours prior to packaging or bottling. Cover with a lid or clean coffee filter or clean paper. Plastic wraps create added condensation and really shouldn't be used. Do not tightly cover an HVAC batch for several hours however, as we are hoping to bleed off any ozone into the room air and up out of the just finished batch.

### The Ideal Colloidal Gold Solution:

Using the HVAC methods and our PUAM (plasma underwater arc method) we want to see is a clear to light pink or rose colored colloidal gold. OLD IDEAS that gold has to turn dark red before its useful are FALSE.

Colloidal gold or 'CG' as we call it, should be produced very slowly and by using the PAUM HVAC method. If you use this method properly, your 32 ounce beaker will heat up during the batch progression, due to the high AC power and also the plasma arc (or little explosions) that the gold electrode tips cause in the batch. As a matter of fact, all HVAC methods create HEAT in your batches and because of this, it is normal to see bubbles form and you may even see steam. Most batches never get above 105 degrees however IF YOU CAN EFFECTIVELY maintain the plasma underwater arc, after about 30-45 minutes, you will be able to discern the light pink color begin to form into the batch. Stirring the batch every few minutes will help the pink hue formulate into the entire batch. You can add a tablespoon of H202 (hydrogen peroxide) to an HVAC batch and the pink tint will occur faster, but it is not necessary for a quality batch.

Please see the HVAC PUAM GOLD chart/ppm strength/amount of pink tinting chart elsewhere in this guide to ascertain our results. Older DC or MHVDC methods can produce a clear colored CG, but can take up to 6 hours and still only raise a few ppm above the baseline of your water (including any additives or starters).

Using HVAC underwater arc methods like ours, you may only see a 2 to 5ppm rise in measurable TDS ranges and yet see a nice pink hue, this is normal, as TDS meters do not register gold nano particles accurately. You may see a pink tint or golden yellow color when pushing your batches past 5 ppm. This does not always occur and you will have to make a weeks worth of batches and log each result to be able to figure your SLP effect and come up with your own baseline, timing charts when dealing with NanoGold production.

Of course, making Colloidal Gold with any DC method is purely experimental and that is why most of our information is based around using HVAC techniques and methods we have created to produce a more consistent result.

Reaching a light hue of pink while making a full 32 ounce beaker of CG, takes about 90 minutes and puts most CG products in the 5 ppm range. Your TDS meters cannot accurately read HVAC particulate liquids. They read about 50% less, on average, because they are not designed to read the smaller NANO particles, rather they are designed to read the micron sized LVDC generated particle and only set to see the harder total dissolved solids.

## Making IONIC GOLD (see 2005-4/05 guides for more)

LVDC generated gold is difficult to produce and is very slow to see any reaction, no matter how high the voltage or current. You may actually SEE the colloidal process happening and maybe some light mist, bubbles and film build-up on the rods, but you may never see a huge increase in PPM on your lab testing meters. This doesn't mean Gold is not forming in the batch, it simply means the meters may not have enough gold or correct calibration to read Colloidal gold effectively.

For slow **LVDC IONIC g**old batches, you may have to try some 'starters' such as a little Colloidal Silver or Gold from a previous batch, this is OK to do for the first time experimenter. Do not add saline's, salts or other additives, however H2O2 can be added at the 1 tablespoon per 32 ounce full beaker rule.

Let your LVDC gold batch progress about 3 to 4 hours and always stop the Gold batch if it starts to change to any color. Your batch may take from 1 to 6 hours to see a 2 to 3 ppm increase over your beginning distilled water baseline. You may actually see the process happening, but the ppm meter readings are low or is not moving, like they do with silver batches. This is normal. PPM meters don't read budding gold batches correctly at first, as they are not calibrated to actually do so.

## Colloidal Color Changes from ongoing batch progression

*Except for PUAM Arc NanoGold, most colloidal color changes that occur are indicative of saturation and particle conglomeration and is an undesirable effect.* This may not matter to NanoGold, but it does matter with silver and other mineral production methods. The particles begin to actually double or triple in size and/or starting to conglomerate. Conglomeration is usually a bad thing and often times hinder a strong COLLOIDAL SUSPENSION for long-term storage or use. These batches also can go into 'RUNAWAY' and turn to brown sludge if not watched carefully.

## 2008 Gold HVAC Method - Plasma Underwater Arc

In about 30-45 minutes you should be getting a warm batch, maybe steamy and the batch should be turning a light pink hue. This is about 3-5ppm and is usually where most producers stop and filter and bottle their gold. It's not necessary to push a HVAC gold batch to red or lavender colors as this is a waste of gold electrodes. The low ppm pink stuff works awesome for arthritic patients and as a mild anti-depressant.

## The Ideal Colloidal Copper Solution

What we want to see is a **CLEAR COLLOIDAL COPPER**, with about 1 to 5 PPM measurement. What we don't want to see is a Yellow or Golden, high ppm Colloidal Copper. Higher ppm readings as well as the yellow color indicates that the COPPER PARTICLES have actually begin to double and triple in size and are most likely conglomerating into large, unsafe to ingest, copper clusters. It is possible to make CLEAR Colloidal Copper up to 10 PPM, but it depends on your SLP effect, lab equipment and purity of the distilled waters your batch began with.

HVAC methods seem to produce higher ppm levels, while maintaining the clear Colloidal Copper. Scientists and Researchers have all gone onto record to state that a GOOD DAILY DOSE of Colloidal Copper is also around 2 PPM. **Colloidal Copper CAN BE TOXIC**, so be careful. It is said that ONE ounce of Colloidal Copper made @ 5PPM, actually equals about 20 regular chelated Copper Supplement Tablets. So be CAREFUL! You can overdose on SILVER, COPPER and GOLD; they are all HEAVY METALS when taken in excess.

Please remember as you attempt your own batch production, because we did not set up your home or business lab and cannot control your lab variables, including SLP effect, PRIDE LABS and the authors and researchers CANNOT GUARANTY THAT YOU WILL MAKE the exact same products as we do here. However, by carefully following our instruction AND writing us about any question that you may have, we promise that your product will come pretty good and probably better than most stuff you can buy pre-made off the web.

## The Ideal Colloidal Zinc Solution

What we want to see is a **CLEAR COLLOIDAL ZINC**, with about 5 PPM measurements. What we don't want to see is a BLUE or Yellow or Golden, Higher PPM Colloidal Zinc. Higher PPM and the BLUE or yellow Color indicates that the Zinc PARTICLES have actually begin to double and triple in size and/or conglomerated into clusters, that NOW reflect LIGHT in the Yellow or Blue spectrum. It is possible to make good, CLEAR Colloidal Zinc up to 10PPM, but it depends on your SLP Effect and Lab equipment and purity of the distilled waters your batch began with. HVAC Methods seem to produce higher PPM Levels, while maintaining the clearer Colloidal Zinc. Scientists and Researchers have all gone onto record to state that a GOOD DAILY DOSE of Colloidal Zinc is about 5 PPM for LVDC productions and 10 PPM for HVAC productions.

## Chaining Batches to produce more

DIGIPRO LVDC power supplies can be 'CHAINED' for double batches at one time. Some units can make up to 10 (TEN) 32oz quarts simultaneously (PS30,PS50,PS75,PS120,PS400). The PS05, PS10 and DUALPORT are limited to 4 total extra chained batches.

Again, recapping, HVAC methods are dangerous as you are using thousands of volts intentionally around water and power cords. HVAC methods <u>can</u> create smaller nano particles which are hundreds of times smaller, than their ionic counterparts. HVAC methods require specialized safety, AC/DC and Chemistry training. HV methods can shock or burn your fingers if not properly handled.

You cannot 'chain' an HVAC batch safely and is dangerous to even attempt it, however, you can usually make 32 ounces maximum per batch in about 1 hour.

The latest HVAC methods are a tad more efficient, and unlike LVDC methods, you don't see the usual oxide and black sediment buildup on electrodes.

## Colloidal Production Equipment & Accessories

Colloidal manufacturing equipment can vary from lab to lab. Basically, the 'known' parameters for industry standard colloidal production for LVDC Ionic liquids are 15-30 VDC and .05 to 250 milliamps. Working with these low of voltages and currents is considered pretty safe, even thought you are working right around water. People are afraid of being shocked and learned at a very young age, water and electricity combined, may be lethal.

With today's UL listed Colloidal Power supplies that are made by PRIDE LABS under the DIGIPRO name, each system (included the HVAC stuff we market) all have Human Ground Fault GFII circuit's built in line with them. This has helped our partners and customers to not report any shock complaints inn over 5 years.

Unfortunately, of the other 12 companies producing AC and DC Colloidal systems, none has a provable UL listing or safety rating like our units do. Now don't get me wrong, I have been shocked plenty of times while setting up and adjusting an ongoing brew session or while trying to adjust 'live' electrodes on one of our HVAC NST systems. You can get quite a jolt from 15 KV @ 30ma!

This is why it is so important that you follow our safety section closely. While we don't recommend doing so, we will show you how to adjust experiments on the fly, even while the high voltage is flying. This is all very dangerous if you don't know what you are doing. In case you screw up and forget your batch is live, the GFII circuits are there acting as a last line of defense, but ultimately, the choice to PRACTICE SAFE MEASURES is entirely up to you.

For HVAC Particulate based liquids, the 'known' parameters start at around 7500 volts AC and go all the way up to 15000 volts AC at between 5 ma to 30 ma.

Results of using 60 or 120 ma power supplies and transformers at HVAC levels, not only has proven dangerous, but really ends up wasting allot of electrode surface unnecessarily. Again, more is not always better in terms of pristine and safe colloidal production.

WHAT'S IN OUR
OUR DIGIPRO
## DELUXE PLUS+ SYSTEMS

CHOICE OF POWER SUPPLY

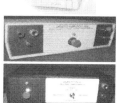

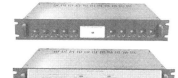

PURE .9999 ELECTRODES
2005 COLLOIDAL PRODUCERS MANUAL
UNDUSTRY STANDARD LEADSETS

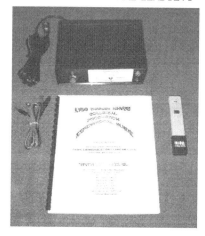

Depending on the method or type of colloidal product you want to produce, you need to get the correct power supply with controlled stationary regulated outputs, so that you will be more able to control your batch progression and brew times.

Unfortunately, there are many 'fly-by-night' colloidal companies that sell inferior systems to people. We have fixed, repaired or traded-up many of their inferior designs, so that the customer could move into a more professional system.

Many of these web designs are pure junk and have loose wires and parts all over the unit. We often have to think that these lay producers MUST have some good luck on their side, as we have not actually heard of too many safety issues or deaths occurring form using these non UL listed generators sold on the web today.

Some Websites sell really bad designs as their Colloidal Generation systems.

PICTURE RIGHT: IS OF A GENERATOR KIT BEING SOLD ON THE NET FOR $75 and requires unhealthy Salt or Saline to make it even work.

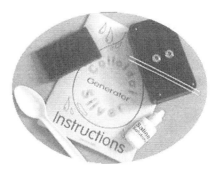

We'd suggest you NOT use battery operated designs and non current regulated units (mostly all the battery operated designs) for LVDC use.

We also suggest that users DO NOT USE MOT (microwave oven transformers) for HVAC uses. We'll explain why, later in the HVAC section. But they are hazardous to your health or anyone close by.

So, besides a good base power supply that is UL Listed, has 3 prong full electrical circuit grounding and is user adjustable, here are the other accessories you ought to have.

## Colloidal Production Lab Items

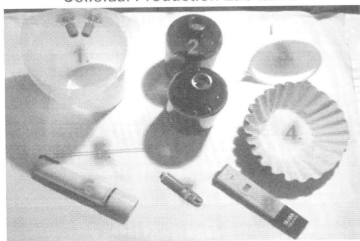

1- Production or Batch container 500 ml to 1000 ml beaker

2- 8 to 16 ounce storage bottles Glass/plastic HDPE

3- Large Plastic or Glass funnel

4- Unbleached paper filters (coffee or better lab filters)

5- Pure .999+ Matched Electrode pair, Silver for making colloidal silver, copper for copper, etc.

6- Small Flashlight (tight beam) for general TYNDALL EFFECT testing. LASER pointer at right is the preferred light device over a flashlight

7- Small red or green laser pointer for full TYNDALL EFFECT batch light testing

8- TSS/PPM Meter for testing baseline distilled waters and for testing particle/ion increase in your colloidal batch to desired ppm outcome.

Now that you have purchased, built or acquired all the items you need, it is time to decide which of the two major methods of Colloidal Production you want to begin with. If you are new to Colloidal Production, you are safest to start out with LVDC equipment and experiments. This type of gear creates the tried and proven 'Industry Standard' Ionic colloidal liquids. Once you get the hang of all the variations of making Ionic minerals, then you can move into the higher powered, HVAC systems and learn how to recreate nano colloidal products.

Hopefully you have read and fully understood the dangers surrounding colloidal mineral production by reading our Safety Section in its entirety. We suggest that your lab techs who will be using the equipment and producing the colloidal mineral products be versed on Electrical Safety measures and they should have passed college course Electronics and Chemistry classes before attempting any HVAC experiments.

## There are actually TWO methods of Colloidal Production

The current Industry Standard method of making silver, copper and zinc is **LVDC IONIC generated method**; this method is used by all GNC, RITEAID and other national Colloidal Silver producers today. It is really an easy method and has been tested for safety many times over and the products have great antiseptic properties. LVDC methods of production is for the BASIC and INTERMEDIATE colloidal producers. The methods are easily recreated in your home or office lab. The second method is the **HVAC PARTICULATE COLLOIDAL METHOD** and is the newest method of production. HVAC methods are open to ADVANCED colloidal producers because they are considered highly dangerous and should not be attempted by new colloidal producers and lab techs.

### DC 'IONIC' BASED PRODUCTION QUICK LOOK

- Easiest method for beginner and advanced commercial or home researchers.
- Tried and proven easy methods for industry standard colloidal production known today.
- Creates a small ionic particle that depending on your lab setup and end strength goal, can be under <.025 micron range for easy bio-availability and absorption.
- This LVDC method is mostly used to create clear colored of silver, copper and zinc colloidal solutions from 1 to 20ppm in strength or light yellow or golden colored strengths in the 15 to 50+ ppm range.
- LVDC systems create a polarized charge on a batch that charges the tiny ionic particle in a natural way and help keep the silver particles in suspension. This charge is aligned with our bodies natural dc charge.
- Shelf life of properly stored finished LVDC products can lat up to 18 months with only a -10-20% drop in efficiency.
- LVDC and HVDC methods have been used successfully experimented with to produce very low ppm clear colored gold, platinum and other minerals.
- The LVDC methods are used to make 16- 32 ounce batches at one time, some DIGIPRO LVDC units can be chained to produce multiple batches at once with the use of extra lead sets and adding the correct amount of production time.
- Most LVDC experiments create a 16-32oz batch of 5 ppm of crystal clear silver, copper or zinc in about 60-90 minutes and about 2 hours for a pure 10ppm single batch..
- LVDC methods use low voltage and low current, making it almost impossible to be shocked or hurt by interfering with a ongoing batch. Some advanced IONIC colloidal researchers are using the DIGIPRO PS120 to experiment with higher voltage dc (up to 120vdc) to produce low ppm gold and platinum solutions.
- Easy to make and easy to keep the pH output for easy absorption on the stomach.
- LVDC IONIC products are the ones currently be carried by Wal-Mart, Rite Aid, GNC and other nationally recognized chains.

### AC 'PARTICULATE' BASED PRODUCTION QUICK-LOOK

- For **Advanced Researchers** who have current lab and electronics knowledge including intimate hands-on experience with LVDC production methods.
- Experimental methods of colloidal production and preliminary lab tests suggest that properly produced HVAC experiments create a smaller (nano-sized) particle, hundreds of times smaller than LVDC systems can normally produce.
- HVAC experiments can be **Dangerous to operate** and if you are not careful, you can get a nasty shock and even get killed if you don't know what safety measures to take. Pride Electronic Labs will only sell these systems to advanced field researchers and producers and they require a liability release signed and accepted before we can ship your HVAC system.
- Infuses a manmade (AC) synthetic charge on each particle to keep it in suspension.
- Longer shelf life than LVDC created batches.
- Particles are not polarized like LVDC systems produce.
- Produces a HIGHLY ENERGETIC charge on each particle, some users actually complain that it infuses them with "too much energy" real world people results are still out on these methods, so any commercial producer will be required to independently test their own methods and samples for safety and use issues.
- HVAC cannot be chained to make multiple batches
- Makes crystal clear Silver, Zinc, Copper and Pink Gold in the 1 to 10 ppm range or greater.
- HVAC NST systems interfere with other lab electrical equipment, computers and TVS, unplug these other devices while a NST Gold batch is going for safety!
- Uses advanced experiments that PRIDELABS includes in their included system manuals such as:

TOTAL SUBMERSION METHOD*
PLASMA UNDERWATER ARC METHOD*

Once you decide on the 'type' of colloidal production style you want use you also have to pick the experiment 'electrode placement method' you want to use.

## For LVDC IONIC or HVAC PARTICULATE MINERALS

The **TSM** (total submersion method) of electrode placement is the most effective and safe method for: Ionic or Particulate Silver, Copper and Zinc

Here is a picture of the TSM method and its common electrode placement. The setup can be as easy as bending electrodes over a lip of a beaker and clamp them securely with alligator clips or by using our QPC-32 ounce batch container with 5-way electrode binding posts built-in. Spacing should be around ¾" to 1" away from each other in a 16 to 32 ounce beaker.

### For HVAC Nano Gold

The PUAM (plasma underwater arc method) has to be employed carefully and requires special safety measures as well as the ability to monitor and slightly adjust gold electrode tips, underwater, while the batch is under full power progression.

The PUAM (plasma underwater arc method) for producing pink or red colored colloidal gold requires a 45 degree glass pipette insulted tube for each gold electrode. The 'ARC BAR' as we call it, sits across the top of the beaker and just the tips of the gold electrodes make semi-contact just barely under the surface of the distilled water.

The gold electrodes need to be insulted by high temp glass pipettes so that maximum voltage and current meet unrestricted at the gold tip ends. When power is applied, the tips either arc in a firey ball of plasma or can literally slap together many times per second, in a sputtering, intentional production arc method.

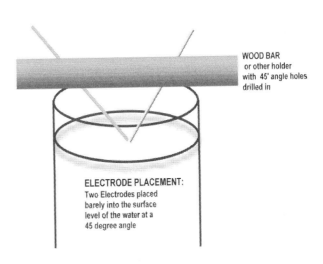

# PLASMA UNDERWATER ARC METHOD
## GLASS BATCH CONTAINER

WOOD BAR
or other holder
with 45' angle holes
drilled in

ELECTRODE PLACEMENT:
Two Electrodes placed
barely into the surface
level of the water at a
45 degree angle

# TSM
# TOTAL SUBMERSION METHOD

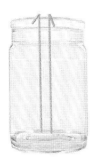

**SECURE BOTH ELECTRODES OVER LIP OF BATCH CONTAINER (BEAKER) BEND OR FORM ELECTRODE TOP (tips) END in a 180 degree BEND, to assist the tops of the electrode to GRAB the LIP securely.**

SPACING FOR HV TSM EXPERIMENTS SHOULD BE ABOUT 1/2" or as CLOSE AS POSSIBLE WITHOUT CAUSING A SHORT OR ARC BETWEEN THE ELECTRODES OR THE ALLIGATOR CLIPS OR LEADS.

To keep the plasma ball arcing, the lab technician is often required to adjust 'hot' or live electrodes or adjust the beaker, leadsets or clamps, during the batch progression of Colloidal Gold, to maintain the all important arc ball. This experiment is not for the faint of heart!

### Distilled Water Notice

Before getting too deep into the actual experiments, the most important thing for any colloidal producer to do is to locate a good source of distilled water. This is where your TDS meter will come in handy for true water baseline testing uses. Buy several gallons of different brands of distilled waters and test each one. Quality water should have a base ppm reading of less than 1 ppm. We have lab tested Arrow Head, Mount Olympus, Albertsons and Safeway brands of distilled water, they usually baseline or "pre-test" out at under 1 ppm, sometimes 000. Most home made distilled water or that which is made fresh from expensive home water distillers, normally test out higher, in the 2 to 10ppm ranges. We suggest keeping it cheap and simple and buy your distilled waters from a reputable store. Most distilled water goes for around $1.29 or less per gallon.

**STAY AWAY FROM BOTTLED WATER, SPRING WATER and distilled water that also says it has been charcoal filtered. True steam distilled water is PURE and needs ZERO FILTERING while making and bottling it.**

Sometimes your distilled water is **_TOO_** pure and because of this fact, the actual colloidal reaction process takes much longer to get going. This is why you need to pick a good water, that is consistent, so that you can make a weeks worth of colloidal batches and log each one, so that you can create your brew time x water ppm=production chart. Once you have done your baseline testing with the water of your choice and have logged down the results, ppm and time, you can create a baseline timing chart that will automatically take in most of your SLP effect.

If you are still having trouble 'starting'; a batch, or the batch sets there for an hour without any ppm change (and you know your power supply and lead sets are active and connected correctly) you can use some H2O2 (teaspoon full for every 32 ounces) or add about 1 ounce of previously made silver to help 'start' the process. This is called 'seeding the batch' and should be done only when forced to do so. Never seed any colloidal batches with salts or saline, as this is how your products can turn toxic and cause your customers to turn BLUE (see Argyria).

## TSM BATCH SETUP

Setup your power supply in an OPEN AREA. You will need a counter or lab space that is at least 36" wide, preferably a wood or other non metallic counter top.

Hopefully your system has a  UL Certification and can be properly grounded. ALL Pride Labs power supplies use UL listed modules and have three prong grounded IEC power cords. Make sure your area is dry to avoid being SHOCKED and always use a 3 prong grounded outlet and a GFII circuit or power strip for safety. DO NOT USE 2 plug to 3 prong plug adapters without running a ground wire. We would suggest you use a GFII plug for best shock protection no matter what!

Make sure your LABWARE (plastic or Glass) is CLEAN and DRY before use to avoid shocks and beginning batch frustrations. Take your batch container, beaker, QPC-32 or new mason jar and set it up in front of you and your power supply. If you already know about power supply leads, test leads, etc, go ahead and hook up the leads to the proper positive (red) and negative (black) power supply ports.

**The polarity does matter in LVDC batches, but <u>DOES NOT MATTER</u> in HVAC experiments.**

Electrodes wear down as the silver or mineral is stripped off them during a batch process. If you always run a batch and the same electrode gets used under the same black lead, than one electrode will get smaller than the other.

You should switch the lead set and swap up the colors all the time, from batch to batch, to keep the wear uniform. HVAC electrodes swap polarity 60 times per second and wear down equally, no matter what color the lead set.

Most of the following steps have to do with LVDC colloidal production; however, there are some notes on HVAC production, so it is wise to read through each LVDC step.

Most likely your PRIDELABS kit did not include the batch container or a QPC-32 and most users in the field already have an idea of what volume of colloidal product they want to produce in any given time frame.

All of our DIGIPRO power supplies and these manuals are designed with the idea that you will be making a 30-31 ounce batch at a time.

Batch containers can be 32oz lab beakers, 16oz glass tumblers, Kerr or Mason quart glass jars, or glass gallon wide mouth jars. Some people are even using a new 12 Cup Coffee Carafe as their batch container. All work great, just remember, the larger the volume, the longer it'll take to produce a batch and of course, some sort of aeration or stirring method should be used.

Whatever container you decide to use, make sure your GLASSWARE is either NEW or at least clean and dry before using them for LAB use. There is a warning that Pride Labs put out to all colloidal producers back in 2002 about using KERR or MASON Glassware.

Most Quart Mason or Canning Jars (even when cleaned) hold a layer of microscopic gunk on/in them as the glass is porous and not lab grade. Sometimes using them over and over again causes Colloidal batches to PLATE OUT and build-up in those pores. Those jars are inexpensive, so make your batches pure by buying a new one. We suggest that you NOT use any plastic batch containers unless they are HDPE approved and you are assured that they will not leech plastic by-products and chemicals into your batches.

### Plastic Lab Beakers

TRI-POUR triangle plastic beakers like the QPC-32 uses, are great for all colloidal batch production but only last about 100 batches. DO NOT wash these tri-pore beakers in the dishwasher as they get hairline cracks.

Next, pick up your alligator clips; you will see a RED and a BLACK Clip. These are POSITIVE (RED) and NEGATIVE (BLACK). **YOUR POWER SUPPLY SHOULD NOT BE POWERED UP AT THIS POINT; it should be in the OFF position during setup.**

Now lets look at the SIDE of the batch container, we will tell you how to place the ALLIGATOR CLIP over the RIM of the GLASS and over the ROD, all at the SAME TIME

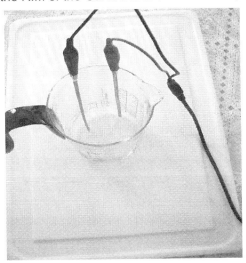

**HINT:** You can bend the end (1") of any electrode 180 degrees (like a tight J) using needle nose pliers and have the bend match your beaker lip. Now take your RED ALLIGATOR CLAMP and PUSH the tabs of the clamp, this opens up the ALLIGATOR CLAMP MOUTH.

Now place **half** of the clamp down over the SILVER ELECTRODE, one side of the JAW goes on the **INSIDE** of the batch container, while the **OUTSIDE** part of the JAW goes on the OUTSIDE of the JAR.

Place these clamps all the way to the HINGE, so that you get a POSITIVELY SECURE ACTION and ELECTRICAL CONNECTION over the SILVER ELECTRODE and the batch container RIM at the same time.

Even though you do this right, it's still possible for the electrode rods to move around or get out of position, so be careful so as not to bump your set up.

Most TSM methods for HVAC and LVDC, suggest that you place the electrodes about 1" part from each other on the side of the beaker. —Any closer and the silver will buildup and conglomerate unnecessarily on the electrodes and can ruin your batch. Too far apart and your batch will never get started.

When not using our QPC-32, many users in the field have come up with homemade ways to better secure the electrode rods into their batch containers; some have used popsicle sticks, boards, clamps, just about anything to secure the electrode wires down into the batch. Just make sure that only the ELECTRODE wire is the only metal or matter actually touching or submerged down into your clean distilled water.

Now do the same thing with the BLACK alligator Clip and SILVER ROD. Position both electrodes perfectly parallel at 3/4" -1" apart inside your batch container. Some ALLIGATOR CLAMPS already came supplied with a BLACK spacer BAR to keep them optimally separated.

Now that you have your connections made at the BATCH CONTAINER SIDE, let's hook up your LEAD SET to the POWER SUPPLY if you haven't done so already. The DIGIPRO SERIES of power supplies use only INDUSTRY STANDARD banana Jacks and sockets.

On your POWER SUPPLY front or rear panel, you will see a red and black banana jack socket or 5 way binding post. You may see a green or third ground socket we will not use for the electrode excitation. You can run a ground wire to an 8 copper ground pipe pounded down into your yard if you want the best ground possible. The RED banana Jack (male) slides into the RED banana SOCKET or BINDING POST hole (female). The same goes for the BLACK. If your POWER SUPPLY has a GREEN or BLUE socket, these are for external grounding and are not used for COLLOIDAL MINERAL PRODUCTION.

If you have a 1-WAY, 2-WAY, 4-WAY or 8-WAY Power PORT Bar, load up the Silver Electrode Pairs and simply plug in the RED/BLACK Leads into the RED/BLACK banana sockets on your power supply. Then simply LAY the ENTIRE BAR across the top of the BATCH CONTAINERS. To load the Silver, Copper or Gold Electrodes: The red/black knobs unscrew to reveal a small vertical hole or shaft where the tip of the electrode attaches. Just place the end into the haft or hole and then finger tighten the RED/Black screw down knobs.

## BOTTOM LOADED POWER BARS w/SPRING CLIPS

If you have spring loaded clip on the bottom of your power bar, insert the STRAIGHT side of the electrode into these spring loaded clips. Check to make sure they are straight, fill your batch container and place the entire rod (with red/blk terminals and electrodes) in the DOWN position and then lay the entire bar across the top of your container.

Power Bars are nice and neat, but they DON'T allow you to place the electrodes closer than .75 -1.00 inches apart. This distance seems to work great for LVDC TSM production methods. If you didn't order the OPTIONAL 1 WAY/2WAY or 4 Way power port bars and/or strips as seen above, please email us and we'll give you a great deal on a port bar.

FILL YOUR BATCH CONTAINER with PURE DISTILLED WATER to about 80-85% full....leave room so the water surface level is about a HALF AN INCH below the alligator clip jaws. NEVER overfill your beaker so that the water is ever touching ANYTHING but the electrodes. Alligator clip metal should NEVER touch the water.

THE FILL LINE is ALWAYS ¾" BELOW the ALLIGATOR CLAMP'S actual METAL, on the batch container. (You **ONLY WANT** the WATER TOUCHING the SILVER, GOLD or COPPER rods, NEVER any other metal, including a metal stirring wand or even the alligator clamps).

Now it's time to double check to make sure your RODS are not TOUCHING EACH OTHER and are in fact PARALLEL to each other inside the batch container. RODS that are touching can produce early POWER SUPPLY failure and even damage, besides the possibility of being shocked. The depth of the rods makes a difference also, make sure that your SILVER RODS or other Colloidal Metal electrodes are not TOUCHING or PUSHING against the BOTTOM of the BATCH CONTAINER - If they are, you may need a taller batch container, **or** simply bend the Silver rods ends out, so that the BOTTOM OF EACH ELECTRODE floats about 1/4 inch up from the bottom of the batch container.

## Grab your PPM Meter and lets take a BASELINE DISTILLED WATER initial reading

Your distilled water should be fairly pure and should read on your PPM meter between 000 through 002 or so. This is your BASELINE distilled water reading. Write it down on your brew time chart or remember it for later.

## Chose your Convection Method and Process

There are two well known methods for good Colloidal Production. They are the **HEAT CONVECTION METHOD** and the standard **COLD (non-convection) METHOD**. The HEAT CONVECTION METHOD is accomplished by heating the DISTILLED WATER to around 120 -135 degrees using a coffee maker to help 'make the batch start' however, heating has been found to be entirely unnecessary with our DIGIPRO higher powered units. Heating the water beforehand simply speeds up the process. Whatever you do, keep your baseline tests consistent. Choose one way and stick to it or you are going to create many batches that become unstable and have odd ppm and color changes.

Just a note: We never heat any waters prior to making a colloidal batch, however, heating does help slower LVDC batches progress faster. There is never a need to pre-heat an HVAC TSM or ARC batch. Use of a separate *new coffee maker is the easiest way to HEAT Distilled water. If you don't have a heat thermometer, let the distilled water heat until you see the wisps of steam come off it. This will be above 120 degrees.  HEATING the distilled water to BOILING point is not necessary.
**HEATING NOTE**

Heating the distilled water is also a natural way to **BRING UP** the natural conductivity of distilled water for 'starting' stubborn LVDC batches.  If you have really **PURE** distilled water, you may want to use the HEAT CONVECTION METHOD to help 'START' your batch without any additives.

The second method is to use the Cold Method. Distilled water stored at ROOM temperature is adequate and the preferred method when your distilled water BASELINE is above 2-5 PPM. Heating also helps stir your progressing batch by use of heat thermals, but the heat thermals only last about 30 minutes or less, as the water cools. DO NOT MICROWAVE YOUR BASE DISTILLWED WATERS. Microwaving the water beforehand destroy and alters the water molecules.  If you are going to use the heat method at all, please use natural heating methods

## START YOUR ENGINES

Now that you have already filled your batch container and installed your electrodes or rods (All you want is the SILVER ROD itself touching the distilled water, NO OTHER probes, electrodes or other metal spoons or stirring devices should EVER touch your pure distilled water WHILE you are producing COLLOIDAL MINERALS) It's time to get going!

PLEASE refer to your INDIVIDUAL POWER SUPPLY OPERATING INSTRUCTIONS to start, adjust and set your Power Supply. If you have a USER ADJUSTABLE lab bench design, like the PS30, PS50, PS75 and PS120, please refer to the CHART on later pages to see your appropriate settings.  Start your batch and plan on at least a 15 to 20 minute run before you power off to dip test your TDS meter for a ppm reading.

## AERATION, STIRRING, BUBBLING and Heat Convection Techniques and hints

All LVDC generated colloidal mineral batches should be stirred or aerated every few minutes or continuously if you want a smaller, evenly distributed Colloidal Particle. Using our AIR PROFILE 1000 aerator/bubbling unit, you can continuously bubble and aerate the batch. Place the SOLID PLASTIC AIR HOSE into your batch. Try not to let it get near the live electrodes and also try not to let the PLASTIC TUBE interfere or accidentally bump or cause inadvertently movement of the pre-set electrodes. DON'T LET THEM SHORT OUT! Using HEATED distilled water can also provide heat convection that can cause a natural stirring effect all by itself. This occurs because of the chemical heat reaction call heat thermals. Most all heated water carries thermals. You may still need to manually stir the batch once every few minutes, just to make sure the SILVER or COLLOIDAL PARTICLE doesn't start to conglomerate or adhere to each other, and form a smoky cloud in your batch container. Use a plastic, glass or wooden spoon to stir your colloidal batch every few minutes, when not using the Pump or other stirring device. It is important to note that while the COLLOIDAL BATCH is in progress, the electrical charge and particles tend to attach themselves to any odd impurities, metals, etc in your batches, so don't leave the spoon or anything else, but the silver rods and possibly the plastic aeration tube, down in a batch while it is turned on.

By now your batch should be started, with the proper voltage and current necessary for the Colloidal Mineral you are producing. Besides stirring and testing the batch, you should not be touching the production, batch container or leads while the power supply is energized. You may not see any of the following occur visibly at first while using a constant Aeration pump, as the turbidity won't allow you to see the COLLOIDAL EFFECT. For your very first colloidal experiment, you may not want to use the aeration unit or heat convection, so that you can see the actual COLLOIDAL LVDC EFFECT progress. You may see wispy clouds of silver particles (LVDC) increase and the batch will actually start to turn light yellow or even golden yellow. A PPM test measurement may show that your batch has progressed over the 10 -15 ppm ranges, when you start to see actual coloring happen. For HVAC methods, you will not see ANYTHING happening in the batch, except that it might bubble and get warm. The reason is that the HVAC method creates such smaller NANO PARTICLES that cannot be seen by the human eye.

During the BATCH PROGRESSION, (you should be stirring the batch - so you will NOT see the silver or brown smoke in an LVDC batch) this smokey cloud is the beginning of COLLOIDAL CONGLOMERATION portion of the batch brew time and if left alone and not stirred, can cause the batch to go into 'runaway' and make a brown, unusable sludge.

### Standard Colloidal Minerals Chart © 2005 by Pride Electronic Labs

| Colloidal Mineral Type | Voltage Ranges | Current Ranges | Batch Times* |
|---|---|---|---|
| Colloidal Silver | 27 - 36 vdc<br>or 2000 - 15000 VAC | 5ma -30ma<br>5ma 1a - 3a Multi-Batches | Depending on your SLP<br>60 minutes = 5-10 ppm LVDC<br>60 minutes = 2-5 ppm HVAC |
| Colloidal Gold | 50 VDC, 90 VDC<br>110 Vdc, 330 VDC<br>10,000 VAC | 35ma, 500ma, 1 Amp or 3 Amps<br>20 Amps | Depending on your SLP<br>90-120 minutes = 2-5 ppm LVDC<br>60- 90  min.= 2-5 ppm HVAC*pink |
| Colloidal Copper & Zinc | 27-32.5 or 50 VDC<br>or 8500-10000 VAC | 5ma, 250ma, 500ma, 1 Amp and 3 Amp | Depending on your SLP<br>45-60 minutes = 5-10 ppm<br>60-120 minutes = 10 ppm |
| Colloidal Platinum | 27-32.5 or 50 VDC<br>or 8500-10000 VAC | 5ma, 250ma 500ma, 1 Amp and 3 Amp | Depending on your SLP<br>45-90 minutes = 5-10 ppm<br>30-120 minutes = 10 ppm |

**We suggest not exceeding the above times** -as with all power supplies, (no matter what design) the colloidal process can possibly create a lot of oxide build-up on the electrodes.

This build-up effect will eventually raise the current and conductivity of the batch sample so high, that the Colloidal Silver Particles conglomerate and your clear sample, might process into a brown SLUDGE (if left totally unattended). To counteract this problem, CLEAN OFF YOUR ELECTRODES between batches if possible. If you do forget to watch a batch and it get conglomerated and goes into a dark yellow or gray color, don't throw it out, you can still filter and dilute it for good plant food. **It really works, A typical Mother's Day Rose stored in the regular vase with Plant food, lasts about 3 to 4 days, the same rose, stored in Colloidal Silver base, lasts 7 to 9 whole days.

OK, now you have made your first batch, but there is still allot to do. When your batch has progressed to your desired or recommended PPM levels as stated above, you are ready to POWER OFF your Power Supply.
Once your unit is TURNED OFF and unplugged for SAFETY, start to dismantle the lead set and electrodes. Remove the electrodes carefully, or you will knock off all the charcoal looking oxide build-up down into your batch.

**Think PURITY HERE FOLKS!**
**Place these on a paper towel for cleaning in a few minutes.**

Next, take your batch container and cover the top and let it settle for 3 to 6 hours in a darkened area, out of sunlight. I would suggest a clean paper towel cover will work to keep dust particles out of your batch. By letting your batches rest, this will assure that any large colloidal particles will fall out of the Colloidal suspension and rest on the bottom of the batch container. Some users let their batches settle for 24 hours.

## FILTERING & DECANTING & STORAGE

You can use double coffee filters (preferably unbleached brown ones) to filter your settled batch. We suggest the first thing you do is decant the pure 99% top level of the Colloidal Liquid into another clean glass container. Then go wash out your batch container and use it for the FILTERED-DECANTED purer Colloidal liquid.

IF you feel confident that your DECANTING METHOD worked, without introducing anything that had settled to the bottom of the batch container, feel free to use a clean funnel to pour your colloidal liquid into your sterilized or clean packaging bottles. These long-term storage bottles should be Amber Glass, Cobalt Blue Glass or HDPE food grade approved, thick plastic white or amber bottles. Seal your bottles with lids and then store in a dry area at room temperature, please keep out of direct sunlight or high heat.

## QUICK STORAGE METHOD

You can use two unbleached (brown) COFFEE FILTERS (Doubled up for purity) to filter your batch right away into your storage container.

This catches most of the large particles and is still very effective and safe to ingest once filtered. When you filter and store the Colloidal Liquid using the QUICK STORAGE METHOD, you MAY get some particle settling.

Well settled, decanted and filtered Colloidal Silver will maintain its electrical charge for months and maintain its antibacterial properties from 12 - 18 months, if stored correctly. Storage in Amber Glass bottles seem to last the longest and shelf life can possibly be extended to 24 months.

## POST MIXING COLLOIDALS to MAKE COMBO'S

You can mix Colloidal Silver and Colloidal Gold into a Storage Bottle for a COLLOIDAL COMBO, as long as the Colloidal Silver and Colloidal Gold were made using the **same LVDC process**. Mix only HV produced methods together, do not mix and match amongst finished products created by different methods.

## CLEAN YOU'RE LAB SUPPLIES:

Lastly, you need to use the scrubbing pad to scrub off the ELECTRODE WIRES, just make them shiny again, Don't worry about making them look new. Also, we suggest that you NOT USE any soap or chemicals to clean your ELECTRODES. Clean you're GLASSWARE for your next batch. REMEMBER, all glassware and electrodes should be cleaned BETWEEN BATCHES!

## LVDC METHOD COLLOIDAL ELECTRODE SWAPPING HINTS:

You will notice that after your batch has progressed to the PPM you want, the CATHODE (Black - Negative) Electrode sometimes gets a dark brown or charcoal coating. This is normal oxide build-up.

We suggest you cleaning the rods after each batch, no matter what. We also suggest to you, that you reverse the Positive (Anode) and Negative (Cathode) electrode all the time, this will help the Colloidal electrode (silver, gold or copper) to be colloidalize at a regular rate.

This way your silver will be evenly ate away  instead of one being full and thick and the other being slim and melted away.  When using the LVDC method, it is REQUIRED that you use TWO SILVER RODS for Colloidal Silver, TWO GOLD RODS for Colloidal Gold and TWO COPPER RODS for Colloidal Copper.

### Gold's Expensive, do I have to buy TWO FULL 24 k rods or wires?
Yes & No, USING HVAC methods, u are required to have two electrodes, but using DC methods, you actually only need one, but it's best to get two up front.

### Here's how to use single LVDC Gold Rods:
Use the single GOLD ELECTRODE as the ANODE or RED-POSITIVE lead for GOLD BATCHES.
For the CATHODE (black) Rod, you can use a silver rod in place of the second Gold Rod. The ANODE is the rod that gets melted away first and actually makes the Colloidal Product

### Colloidal Combo's?
Some users experiment with a Gold/Silver Anode Cathode production. They reverse the LEAD POLARITY to make Colloidal Gold for 5 minutes and then alternate and make Colloidal Silver for the next 5 minute period. They keep alternating the leads at the Power Supply side back & forth to create some very healthy and unique Colloidal Combinations.

### Storage Container Hint:
You can use AMBER/BLUE glass bottles or even the newer HDPE APPROVED FOOD GRADE WHITE PLASTIC CONTAINERS. Glass always stores the CS Longer, by about 25 to 30 percent. Plastic is the Next best storage, but make sure it's not regular PET plastic bottles.

# HVAC NANOPARTICULATE COLLOIDAL PRODUCTION PRIMER & EXPERIMENTS
## This information is intended for the use by advanced and experienced colloidal researchers only

PRIDELABS.US, its owners, officers, employees or the authors of this Information cannot warranty, guaranty or promise that you will be able to effectively re-create ANY OF THE experiments contained in this manual.

Using High Voltage AC power supplies can be potentially hazardous and because of this PRIDELABS takes no responsibility for your use of this kit. We also are not responsible for any legal or medical complaints/issues arising out of your use of this experimental information. This guide is presented as an informational tool only and should be construed as such. YOU SHOULD HAVE FIRST OBTAINED and READ THROUGH OUR LIABILTY RELEASE AND DISCLOSURE FORM signed it and returned it to PRIDELABS.

It is assumed you have some prior lab knowledge in Chemistry, Electronics and/or biology experience and by purchasing and placing together this kit, you assume all liability in the event of injury or even death while using this kit or information. Because this kit comes partially un-assembled, it is legally sold and marketed as a kit ONLY.

Please keep this kit and all components out of the reach of untrained users, children and teens. You can be SHOCKED or KILLED by HIGH VOLTAGE ELECTRONIC DEVICES! There are several important benefits to using HVAC/HVDC over LVDC methods to produce Colloidal Silver, Gold, Copper, Zinc and Platinum liquids; they are listed below:

**1- Purity:**
A properly produced HV (high voltage) batch makes the colloidal product somewhat faster and virtually without any by-products on the actual electrodes. Not only do you **not** get allot of electrode buildup, you may not even have to wipe down or scrub your electrodes in-between batches like you have to do with Ionic batches. You will also produce a pure, pristine colloidal batch. We always suggest that no matter how pure your created batch becomes that you post batch decant or filter your batches. High Voltage processes also eliminate most of the run-away effect and conglomeration that LVDC batches suffer from.

**2- Particle Size:**
Using the correct High Voltage methods, you can achieve a proven & smaller **nano sized particle** of whatever metal you are trying to produce. LVDC methods result in particles and ions in the much larger **micron range.** .

PARTICULATE NANO-PARTICLES are difficult for a standard TDS or PPM meters to read accurately. Unlike the IONIC (LVDC created) minerals, where an off the shelf TDS/PWT PPM meter can read the conductivity and calculate fairly accurate PPM totals, an HVAC batch creates a much smaller, less conductive (metallic) particle, that normal TDS/PPM meters cannot accurately read.

Sometimes a simple visual test of color, hue or Tyndall line effect or set timing based upon known outside lab tests, is needed to estimate strengths of HVAC produced batches. Some researchers actually attempt to vaporize a certain amount of gold as an example, into the batch. For instance, one researcher on the Colloidal Gold Yahoo group offers the idea that 1 mm of gold wire, 22 gauges, vaporized into a 16 ounce batch equals about 100ppm of colloidal gold. We assume that he has paid for and received a certified outside lab result to come up with this result.

Regular labs that were once used for testing LVDC created (micron-sized IONIC CS products) simply will not be able to estimate the nano-particle size and true micrograms of silver or other mineral (and PPM) without expensive electron scanning microscope and other advanced testing. See the Colloidal Gold color/timing charts included at the end of the Colloidal Gold section to see our outside lab results.

### 3- Production Times:

Using High Voltage (depending on the method used) some production times go down and volume can go up simultaneously. The high voltage TSM (Total Submersion Method) is slowest, while the CONE method is faster and the PAM UNDERWATER ARC method is the fastest production method that PRIDELABS has tested to date.

### 4-Concentration:

As stated above, the amount of PPM per concentration rates can be more effectively created and higher PPM amounts are not unheard of. No longer do you have to settle for 2-5ppm of clear, LVDC created colloidal mineral, you can easily push your batches and finished product into actual 5-20ppm (or more) concentrations using some of our methods.

### 5- Shelf Life:

Most HV produced Colloidal Products are said to have an indefinite shelf life, however, we have only stored and tested Nano-Particulate Colloidal Minerals for about 2 1/2 years. All colloidal liquids should be therefore stored in glass bottles (amber preferred) or solid white or amber HDPE plastic containers. We have also tested properly stored glass batches up to 2 years, without any ppm drop or fallout. We have also tested HDPE plastic stored batches for up to about 18 months, without any drop in ppm or fallout measured.

Quick overview of our experiments:

IF YOU ARE MAKING COLLOIDAL MINERALS to RESALE, your local health department may require your lab to be certified before production can happen. You must also follow all state, local and FDA/FTC DSHEA regulations before selling any finished products.

### _LAB ALERT!!!_

RF INTERFERENCE NOTE - _ALL HV EXPERIMENTS and the PAM create SOME MAJOR electrical interference to nearby electrical devices, TV's and Radios. Even computers are susceptible to interference and even damage._

_HV EXPERIMENT'S SHOULD NOT BE ATTEMPTED by anyone with a PACE MAKER or near medical life support devices within 75 foot radius and even in your same household. The actual PLASMA ARC that occurs is like a transmitter and it will create STATIC on nearby radios and TV sets and any medical devices in the room. EVEN IF YOUR TV or RADIO is turned OFF, do not LEAVE THEM CONNECTED to the same electrical outlet that the PS15, PS100, 200 or PS1000 are connected to. You can blow out, damage or destroy ANY ELECTRICAL DEVICE that shares the same plug of AC circuit with an HV POWER SUPPLY._

## PLASMA UNDERWATER ARC METHOD
### GLASS BATCH CONTAINER

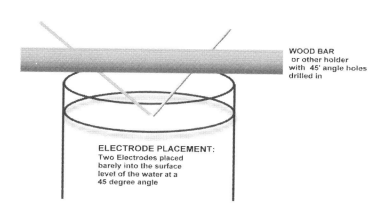

WOOD BAR
or other holder
with 45' angle holes
drilled in

ELECTRODE PLACEMENT:
Two Electrodes placed
barely into the surface
level of the water at a
45 degree angle

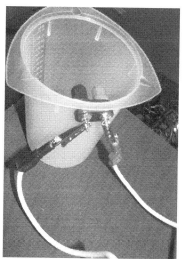

# THERE ARE REALLY ONLY <u>TWO STABLE HVAC</u> EXPERIMENTS YOU SHOULD ATTEMPT:

## HIGH VOLTAGE AC PAM-u (PUAM)  Plasma Underwater Arc Method

## TSM  Total Submersion Method

**TSM ™ (Total Submersion Method)** For Nano Silver, Copper, Zinc (not gold) and other minerals

This is the regular 'LVDC LIKE' method used for 30 years to make LVDC Silver. This is the old 'standby' method where the researcher totally submerges both electrodes into the batch container, separated by an appropriate distance. This method used at HV is the slowest of all HV Colloidal Production Methods. The TSM method also takes the longest to create and your batch will actually began to 'hat-up' as the plasma energy is beginning to disperse into your distilled water batch container. Use of an aeration tube and/or constant stirring will help keep the batches temperature down and also disperse the particles throughout the batch more efficiently. This method also

**PCM ™ (Plasma Cone Method)** For Nano Silver, Copper, Zinc (not gold) and other minerals

Not quite the PAM (Plasma Arc Method) but close to the TSM. The PCM uses the water and creates an actual vortex or 'cone' that rises up and touches the rod, even if it is hovering well above the surface of your base distilled water level. The cone also swirls around the electrode rod at a fast pace and using a laser pen or bright spotlight flashlight, you can see the tornado effect happening. This method focuses the energy at the point of the hovered electrode and is good for systems that are rated under 10kv and 10ma output. Most NST's or modern day lab supplies for HV use, just can't maintain the voltage and current necessary to maintain a full TSM or full PAM, this is the "cheating" way to minimize current 'drag down' on smaller systems, while maintaining full voltage and current at the electrode tip..

**PAM-u (Plasma Arc Method-underwater)** For Nano Gold and possibly experimentation in Silver, Copper, Zinc and other minerals

This is the best method for making colloidal gold. Faster then the TSM method, with a properly set up PAM-u experiment, you can make a light pink colloidal gold, rated at about 5 to 10ppm in about 60-90 minutes, based upon a quart batch container.

Created back in 1998, by the Pridelabs Research Team, the PAM-u is one of the more reliable ways for a field researcher to actually recreate industry standard pink or reddish colored Colloidal Gold. You can arc vapor most any mineral, including silver, but use of the PAM is not suggested for anything but gold at this time.

If you use the PAM for other minerals, let us know about your results, we would be interested in seeing how you did it and what the outcomes were. We have researched other minerals using the PAM and got different and sometimes odd outcomes. To setup a PUM, you will need a 45 degree angled glass Insulated pipette bar, see picture below. The glass pipettes are 3" long, so we suggest that you buy a minimum of a matching pair of 4 to 6 inch long 24 k gold wires.

The purpose of the pipettes is to act as an electrode insulator and FOCUS the arc at where the electrodes almost touch. 18 to 22 gauge wire tips conduct the underwater arc fairly easy, all without melting the end of the wire tips. Some melting will always occur at some point, so don't be alarmed, when your gold tip ends form a little gold bulb. If you can make pink or red gold without the melting, more power to you!

Research using thicker rods or larger diameter electrodes doesn't seem to make the process run faster, in fact, it actually makes most NST systems see a bigger short potential and the Ground Fault circuitry actually reduces the NST output by up to 70%. Smaller is cheaper and sometimes easier on the NST equipment.

## THE PUAM PIPETTE BAR
The bar simply lies across the top of the batch beaker or batch container.

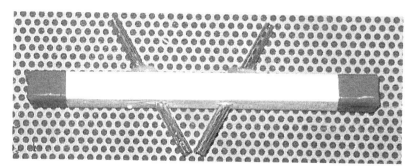

To better sturdy the bar, you can use a clamp of other equipment to temporally secure the bar from moving about.

LEFT: Here is an actual PUAM gold experiment. The bar lays across the beaker and the researcher fills the beaker with barely enough distilled water to reach the bottom few centimeters over the galls tube ends. The gold electrodes are slid down inside each pipette and secured at the other end or top, by the HV power supplies Lead alligator clips.

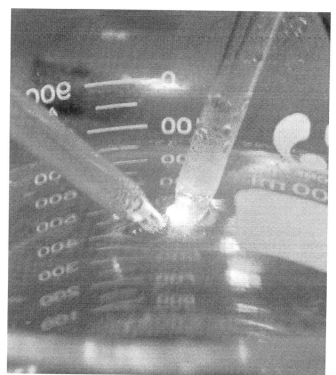

The tips of the gold electrodes need to be almost touching and positioned barley under the surface of the water.

This allows the gold tips to almost touch and when HV power is applied, the gold tips conduct and throw a blue white underwater arc between one another. The main purpose of the PUAM is to expertly position and baby-sit the electrode position so that a continuous arc is maintained.

A small arc or a large arc all creates the same effect. It sinters off nano particulate chunks of pure sub atomic gold in every arc explosion. These explosions are happening at least 60 times per second and more.

GETTING THE ELECTRODES SET PROPERLY AND ALLOWING THE ARC TO PROGRESS IS THE MOST DIFFICULT MANUEVER. UNLESS YOU ARE USING PLASTIC PLIER OR OITHER GLASSWARE, NEVER ATTEMPT TO ADJUST THE ARC, PIPETTES OR HV LEADS/ALLIGATOR CLIPS WITH THE HV POWER ON.

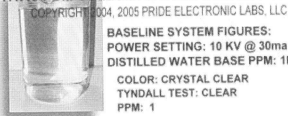

# HVAC PCM COLLOIDAL GOLD DENISITY CHART

**BASELINE SYSTEM FIGURES:**
**POWER SETTING: 10 KV @ 30ma**
**DISTILLED WATER BASE PPM: 1PPM**

COLOR: CRYSTAL CLEAR
TYNDALL TEST: CLEAR
PPM: 1

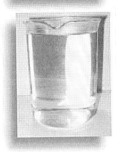

TIME INTO BATCH: 30 min
COLOR: Light Hue
TYNDALL TEST: Very light
PPM: 1.2

OUTSIDE LAB
RESULT ON THIS
SAMPLE WAS: 2.5ppm

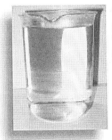

TIME INTO BATCH: 68 min
COLOR: Light pink hue
TYNDALL TEST: Light
PPM: 1.8

OUTSIDE LAB
RESULT ON THIS
SAMPLE WAS: 4.5ppm

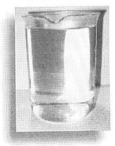

TIME INTO BATCH: 80 min
COLOR: pink hue
TYNDALL TEST: Light
PPM: 2.0

OUTSIDE LAB
RESULT ON THIS
SAMPLE WAS: 6.85ppm

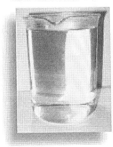

TIME INTO BATCH: 100 min
COLOR: pink to light red
TYNDALL TEST: thicker
PPM: 2.2

OUTSIDE LAB
RESULT ON THIS
SAMPLE WAS: 10ppm

COLOR INDICATION ABOVE IS slightly
exhaggerated & averaged
for use on Color & Grayscale Printers

Some batches progress from clear to reddish or pink tint after about 45-60 minutes and the water heats itself in about 20 minutes to around 130-150 degrees, so be careful when pouring or decanting.

Real Colloidal Gold of any measurable ppm strength should have a light pink hue, or even a reddish tint.

Making dark red colored gold requires that your batch beaker or container be smaller around 4 to 8 ounces. It takes a smaller batch container and longer brew times to produce red gold.

There is also a point of saturation when the gold particles hit a certain level and begin to conglomerate and cause the darker red hues or even violet or purple colored batches.

We suggest that you stick with the methods and experiments we describe and stop your gold batches at or under <10 ppm or light pink in color.

### What is happening at the Plasma Arc Level

The electrode tips are actually moving back and forth, in a 60 cycle sputtering method and with each short, the HVAC causing a baby explosion or arc and sinters off the nano gold particles in a bubble of pure plasma.

This process creates the colloidal gold. Of course there is a more detailed, scientific reason about an atom losing an electron, etc, but the method easily creates a tried and proven low ppm colloidal gold.

**PPM or TDS Meters don't read Nano Particulate particles normally, some PWT meters do however**

As we told you earlier, most HVDC and HVAC methods produce highly particulate particles, which do not measure the same as particles produced in the IONIC range of LVDC produced batches.

Most handheld TDS/PPM and uS meters made by Hanna and others are meant for water testing and cannot accurately measure true particulate amounts in an HVAC batch.

To help you identify and estimate your Nanogold strengths of each batch, we sent many HV produced batches to an independent, outside lab and we produced this Visual Color Chart to help guide you in making HV produced particulate colloidal minerals.

Your results can vary and we do not offer any accuracy in your batch outcomes, so you may want to have your own methods and experiments checked by your own independent lab to be sure.

You can use the HVA chart below as a basic guide for making a 1000ml (32 oz) batch in a given time, without needing to measure and test ppm in most circumstances.

*Site Location Probabilities will affect this out come by plus/minus 5-10%

The PPM results indicated in the chart are what a an outside lab stated our strengths were. The "SAMPLE PPM" level listed is what a typical Hanna Labs TDS meters read in our lab.

The color is fairly accurate; the dark pink was about 2.2 ppm over a starting baseline of 000 for the distilled water used in our testing.

Timing Chart - Batch Size Method

| COLLOIDAL MINERAL | METHOD USED | TIME to PRODUCE 32oz | HANDHELD TDS/PPM METER FINAL READING | OUTSIDE LAB RESULT |
|---|---|---|---|---|
| Gold | PAM-u | 90 min | 3-5ppm +/- 10% | 6.1 ppm +/- 10% |
| Gold | TSM | 14 hours | 5-7ppm +/- 10% | 2.9 ppm +/- 10% |
| Gold | PCM or TCM (cone) | 3 hours | 2.1 ppm +/- 10% | 1.8 ppm +/- 10% |

**LET'S GET GOING ON AN UNDERWATER ARC METHOD:**

Start by filling your BATCH CONTAINER about 80% full; leave the water level about 1" below the lip of the container.

Leave room for your Alligator clips or the bottom part of the 45 DEGREE HV Pipette bar, just make sure the alligator clips or HV wires are close to the water, or they may act as ELECTRODES and arc towards the water surface level, a BIG NO-NO. If it means only filling your container 70% full, then do so.

*MAKE sure the alligator clips are snug over and making as much contact to the top of the electrode as possible. If you are getting a sizzling sound or seeing electrical arcs from under the alligator clips, your clips are not making SURE CONTACT, you should re-attach them to form a MORE SURE CONNECTION to your electrode wires.*

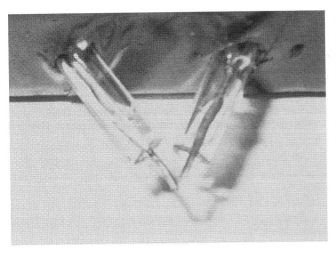

Using the pipette bar is where you set up your tips as shown in the pictures above. You adjust the gold electrode wires down into each pipette, with just the tips poking out through the open bottoms of the pipettes.

Get the electrodes spaced just close enough where they will maintain a continuous spark or arc, without shorting out and sticking to each other.

Alligator clips hold the top of the electrode above the pipette tube. Secure, tape or use other holding equipment may be necessary on the top of the pipettes, where the electrode wire is being clamped to.

Moving the alligator clips even slightly can cause the arc to stop or the electrode tip under the water, to weld together, so be careful adjusting a live batch or even a batch on standby. Make sure you are using plastic kids screwdriver or plastic children's pliers to adjust the clamps, electrodes or pipettes on an live powered batch.

Barely fill the distilled water level so that the arc happens just barely under the surface of the water. Too far down into the water and you will ground out the batch and won't be able to maintain an arc. The goal here is to   maintain a continuous arc without having the electrode short out and stop the process.

This is where you arc will form if set up correctly. If the tips are too close water surface, the arc will grab the water and pull it up to and around the tip of the anode, this becomes the PCM (c**one**) method, not the PAM we really want.

If this 'coning' happens after you energize your power, your anode tip end is too close to the surface level. You will have to de-energize your power supply (turn it off as mentioned in this chapter) and simply BEND the tip out or up a little more so that the tip end is a tad farther above the surface of the water level, then re-energize and you'll see the plasma arc lightening bolt start to form.

Of course if you have a safe plastic or wood tool, you can use it to adjust the anode bend or tip end slightly while energized, but use caution and do a live experiment adjustment at your own risk. All of our Electrodes are about 6" long, however, when using the PAM arc method, you really only need a few inches.  If you have to, you can bend the electrode into any form that will work, we only give you examples. The actual 'bending' is up to you.

** The reason we want the PLASMA ARC to form on **just the TIP or END** of your electrode is because the PLASMA ARC forms easier and with LESS ACTUAL power, making it safer for long term operations of your PS15k or PS200 or your NST.

At this minimum level, the unit *IS PRODUCING* high voltage and even though it's not a lot, you can be slightly shocked and you may feel a 'tingle' if you try to adjust the wires or electrodes without using any INSULATED adjustment tools.

If you are comfortable that you have your Electrodes bent and in place and have you water level where you think it should be, go ahead and start to turn up the HV LEVEL, just a little bit at a time,  until you actually see the little PLASMA ARC or LIGHTENING BOLT form **and stay** on continuously.

**THIS IS VERY** unnerving for the first time, but the pop, sizzle, water movement, little blue arc forming, is ALL NATURAL. The ARC is pretty cool at first and it may startle you a little, you cannot be shocked or harmed by this little natural lightening bolt as long as you DON'T TOUCH IT!

<u>WARNING</u>

Make sure your FOREARMS are not laying on the desk or along side any LEADS or WIRES, you could be shocked slightly, even touching the insulted lead HV wires during a PLASMA charge may slightly shock you. This voltage is so low, that it may feel like a tingling, but it's still unnerving and not fun.

The power supply cannot be safely used for actual human attachment, like some other medical low power tens units. The PS15 and PS100 put out about 1000 times more power and can cause nerve damage, shock or even death when making prolonged contact with its output.

For adjustable power supplies:
Once the PLASMA ARC has formed, turn **DOWN** the HV LEVEL until the Plasma Arc almost stops. If you turn it too far and it fails, just quickly turn back up the VOLTAGE OUTPUT LEVEL knob until it forms again, and then leave it there. Once you have it adjusted for **MINIMUM**, your HV power supply should NOT get hot, however, YOU WILL SMELL electrical ozone being created as it brews your batch, you may also see steam and bubbles form on your glassware, and this is NORMAL.

## TRICKING YOUR GOLD BATCHES TO BEHAVE BY "SEEDING"

Gold is a permeable and rather stubborn mineral to get to sinter off an electrode, even under the arc process. To help push a gold batch into sintering, you can add two drops of Hydrogen Peroxide to a 16 ounce beaker or 4 to 6 drops into a 32 oz beaker to help "start" the process. This will quicken the batch heating time and you will see the pink or reddish colored gold begin to hue after about 30 minutes. You don't have to "trick" a batch if you would rather not.

Another trick is to seed your batch with some colloidal silver. Add 1 oz of 5 to 10ppm silver to a 16 ounce batch, or 2 ounces for a 32 ounce batch. This adds a bit of antiseptic properties to your gold batches as well.

<u>Never use salt or saline's to "push" any colloidal batch.</u>

For GOLD BATCHES, progressing the batch brew time may increase the PPM, but, some researchers have found that Gold plateaus at a certain point and attempting to push the batch by longer brew time, results in a flat reading and meters may actually start to reverse. What this means, is that on a given day and time, gold can sometimes stop at 2ppm or get pushed past 5ppm etc and no matter how long you attempt to let it brew past that 'plateau point' it's PPM increase in negligible.
There is no set rhyme or reason to creating Colloidal Gold, there are many ways to experiment with it, but it always seems to get to a certain level and stops. Some researchers have stated they have been able to push their gold batches to a light purple or light red coloring, every researcher who did this had to add a stabilizer, such as salt, saline's, etc…which (even with gold) we feel it is not a good idea.

Whenever you add saline's to gold, it will always create unwanted gold chloride as a by product. The same thing can be said of creating Colloidal Silver batches.
Every production method discussed in this guide final batch ppm outcome can see it's final ppm rating drop by up to 50%, it's always good to let all finished batches stand for 24 hours and if you are attempting to get a final 3PPM reading, we'd suggest that you brew the batch up to about 6PPM, and then let it stand covered for 12 to 24 hours.

## If you are HEARING NOISES, smelling OZONE or seeing smoke

If you are hearing a sizzle or see arcs that occur at the ALLIGATOR CLIPS (where they attach over your electrodes), you should POWER DOWN your unit and use SAFETY PRECAUTIONS, such as DECHARGING your unit. Once powered down, use a plastic, non-insulated tool and try to re-position your alligator connections over your electrode wires for a much firmer contact. The ONLY PLACE YOU WANT TO SEE ANY PLASMA ARC is between the ELECTRODES TIPS underwater, never anywhere else.

Alligator clips should not SMOKE/SIZZLE or get hot enough to melt the RED or BLACK plastic rear caps on the alligator clamps if they have been put on correctly enough to make a good HV connection. The CLIPS should be securely clamped over the electrodes and actually **BITE INTO** the electrode top bend or lip of the glass batch container. Using the Arc Bar, just clip the alligator clamps on the exposed gold electrode just barely above the rim of the glass pipette.

Sometimes clipping the alligator clip at an **angle** instead of straight up and down over the top of the electrode will be needed. There's NO CLEAR RULE on securing the electrode, just make sure they are connected securely against the electrodes.

We have tried for years to come up with an easier **'set it and forget it'** electrode holder, but because of the voltages and temperature that the electrodes heat to, most everything we have experimented with, such as a wooden block, adapter or single clamp, have failed after several uses when using unpredictable High Voltage power. The only thing that works easily, is the 45 degree arc bar.

Because of this, we would love to hear from field researchers, such as yourself, about how you are dealing with this problem. If you come up with a usable alternative and we can reproduce them, we will each idea in our manuals and systems and give you credit for them and any drawings or pictures you send us.

## PCM EXPERIMENT

(Next to Slowest HVAC Method) Total or Plasma Cone Method
To experiment with the **PCM (Cone Method)** you should submerge the cathode (black) lead with proper electrode down into the batch container as shown. You can use the pipettes or just your electrodes bent at converging (but not touching) positions. Once this is secure with the alligator clamp holding it firmly in place on the lip or rim of your batch container, you can move onto the ANODE (red or HOT) electrode placement. This gets a bit tricky here and there is VERY LITTLE DIFFERENCES in the CONE and ARC methods here.

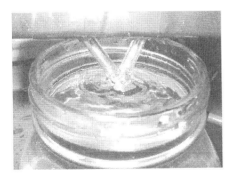

Fill your batch container about 90% full, leaving you about 3/4 of an inch from the rim of your glass to the surface level of the distilled water. Bend your ANODE (RED) Electrode as seen in the Illustration on page one. Make the **END or TIP** of the electrode slightly hover above and/or barely touch the surface of the water. Move your hands away and temporarily apply HV power.
Watch the water around the end of the ANODE electrode, it should attempt to 'CONE-UP' or travel UPWARDS to the electrode and up its shaft about a few millimeters. You can easily see this occur with the naked eye.

It will create a VORTEX or UPSIDE DOWN CONE around the electrode wire. You may also see a vortex form around the cathode electrode that is submerged, this will occur near the surface area of the water, where that electrode is initially submerged. Use a laser pen or bright flashlight and you will see a natural occurring vortex occurring around and about the coned up water. The particles are swirling around at hundreds of miles and hour; you will actually see the sparkles fly by as it creates them.

Remember, the PAM (Plasma Arc Method) is set up exactly like the Cone method above, but requires you to place the anode electrode further above the water, so that the actual water cannot reach or 'cone up' to reach the Anode Electrode tip, but rather because of the increased distance, it will actually create a PLASMA ARC or small continuous SPARK of lightening. This is tricky to maintain, and requires setting the electrode an EXACT DISTANCE from the surface of the water.

**QUESTION: I find that trying to ADJUST the anode (red or main) electrode is tricky, and I think it would be easier to actually turn on the HVAC output and adjust the distance between the electrodes in the water, while the unit is ON, Is it possible to adjust the ELECTRODE PLACEMENT WHILE THE HVAC IS GOING?**

**YES**, but do this at your OWN RISK and you MUST use some sort of plastic pliers, clamp or other wooden non-metallic device to push around the electrode anode. Try and slightly move or nudge the anode electrode or at least try to move it just enough to create the PLASMA ARC, or bolt of plasma.
►**Make sure any tools you are using are plastic or wood and contain NO METAL parts, or you will receive a jolt**

**A Few more Production & Use Questions: I made a double batch of 'chained' Colloidal Silver and 20 minutes into the batch, I tested both samples with my PPM meter and the batch on the left was at 11 ppm and the batch on the right was at 12 ppm, Why the difference?**

Electrodes that are not exactly parallel to one another, even by a centimeter, can cause the process in one batch to progress faster or slower than a batch right next to it. Sometimes one lead set is connected more securely and making a better electrical contact to the electrodes. This is normal to get a variable batch when chaining.

**Question about Silver Oxide Build-up: I want to make 10 ppm batches and I notice that the Anode or Cathode electrode gets a dark silver build-up on it before the batch reaches 10 ppm, it's making charcoal particles float off into my batch, what should I do?**

You can temporarily stop the batch, and wipe down the electrodes and re-insert them into the batch. You can also make less than 10ppm silver batches, which produce a smaller particle, without the heavy build-up.

People think that more ppm is better, in fact, the higher the ppm, the larger the particle, this is especially true when making yellow or golden yellow batches. As stated before, our lab tests PROVE that you are getting a more pristine, smaller particle production, when you stop your batches well before the color change. Yellow is indicative of a larger particle batch, always. Clear is always BEST!

## ACCESSORIES

If you purchased the DELUXE KIT with air, you may have an optional PROFILE 1000 Aeration (Air Pump) unit, with 18" of tubing and a 6" plastic or glass rigid insertion tube/clamp set. This allows CONSTANT AERATION, OXYGENATION and STIRRING, to produce even smaller, EVENLY dispersed colloidal particles. We use silicone and trouble-free tubing and are silicon based and you should replace any bad tubing with a like product. Use of the aeration unit is not always necessary when making clear, 10ppm or under CS, but is included for your aeration experimentation.

## QUICK AERATION UNIT SETUP

The Aeration or stirring aquarium pump and 18" hose, simply plugs into any 110 VAC ONLY outlet. Place the hose down in some portion of the BATCH CONTAINER (opposite side of the electrodes preferably) you are making your CS in. Try NOT to let the hose interfere with the SILVER ELECTRODES. The hose is big and can sometimes push against the rods, causing them to short out. The rods should always be kept about 3/4 " to 1" apart. Use of the Aeration Pump adds continuous stirring and aerating the batch, so the Silver electrodes won't build up Silver Oxide and you won't have to clean the electrodes on a heavy CS production day.

**NOTE:** If your Electrodes are turning charcoal or black, there is build-up of Silver Oxide, if your batch has not reached you preferred PPM level yet, you might find it necessary to stop the BATCH and wipe of or use the scour pad to scour the electrodes. If you MAKE less than 15 PPM, the electrodes SHOULD not be blackened to the point of having to clean them during a batch. ALL ELECTRODES should be wiped down after EACH individual Batch and prior to their NEXT use.

## TESTING YOUR BATCHES

Let's learn about your **BASE LINE TESTING** and **HOW TO USE the TDS/PPM Meter**:

All Deluxe DIGIPRO Kits come with a Milwaukee, HM Labs or Hanna Instruments Brand TDS-1 Handheld Meter.

These meters are fairly accurate for testing the purity AND/OR the PPM of water, including Colloidal SILVER.

Hanna also makes the LAB PWT desktop PPM meter. The Circuitry and testing measures in the handheld TDS-1 meters are similar to the more expensive PWT Desktop meters. PWT Meters are between 75.00 and 130.00 for most models, the LAB PWT Desktop unit is closer to one thousand dollars.

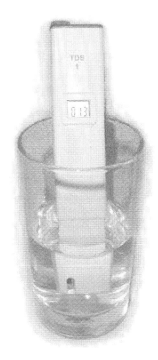

Our Engineer found that we could easily and fairly accurately re-calibrate the TDS-1 meters to equal (within 2 ppm accuracy of the PWT BENCH LAB meter.

We have tested our TDS-1 CS Calibrated meters against PPM meters that cost thousands of dollars and come very close to the readings on a given sample batch. Your TDS-1 meter can also measure Colloidal Gold, Copper and other minerals, but not as accurate as silver. All PPM Meters from Pride Labs come calibrated for actual ppm readings of Water and Silver only.

**BATTERY REPLACEMENT:**
Your PPM Meter has a top lid (usually black, containing unit's power switch). This lid can be popped off to reveal 4 small batteries. **If your meter ever starts reading funny characters or going dim enough or starts reading very low ppm readings or when you can only see it at a certain angle, your batteries may need to be replaced.**

Radio Shack carries these batteries and they will most likely install them for free, if you ask. Under the lid is a short 1" red/black wire, BE CAREFUL WHEN REMOVING LIDS, don't stretch or break the delicate wires.

## Checking and Working on your TDS Meter:

Let's take a **BASELINE READING** of the new distilled water you are going to use: if you haven't already done so, pour distilled water up to about 80-85% full in your batch container, remember you will have to leave room for alligator clamps or power port clamps.

Now take the bottom cap off of your TDS meter, set it aside.

See how far up the cap goes from the bottom of the TDS meter? About 1.75" max, **NEVER DIP THE METER INTO** any LIQUID **past** the bottom **1.75" of the TDS Meter**, the water can reach the CIRCUITRY and **RUIN THE METER**.

REMEMBER: only the BOTTOM third half goes down in the water inside your batch CONTAINER - ever! Turn on the **TDS** meter power switch, the meter LCD readout will read 000 (zero zero zero).

Place the meter down into your water as described in the above paragraph. Let the meter temperature compensate for about 10-30 seconds. The meter will settle pretty much on the same figure. Let's say it settles on 003 ppm. That is your BASELINE and tells you how PURE your DISTILLED WATER is. Write down or remember this figure. You'll need it later when figuring out your true PPM at the finish line.

### BATCH  TDS / PPM METER ALERT NOTE:

USE the TDS submersion technique you just learned to properly test your batch as it progresses. Be careful NOT to test your batches under power. TDS meters DO NOT READ ACCURATELY while there is HVAC or LVDC VOLTAGE GOING to the Silver Rods. ALWAYS TURN OFF or unplug your power supply while doing a 30 second PPM test.

### IF I CAN'T ACCURATLY TEST the HV BATCH with my TDS/PPM Meter, how will I know I'm actually making anything?

The pictures below shows the tyndall line laser testing result. Part of the reason we wanted to show you this picture is because it shows an actual TYNDALL EFFECT. See how you can SEE the BEAM of the flashlight inside the water? It's a CLOUDY BEAM running from left to right.  There should be no big sparkles seen in the beam of light. When you look at your batch without a beamed of light, It should be pure and clear.

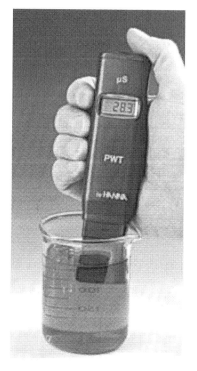

A new glass of distilled water will pass the light beam clear through, you will not see the beam in the water. The light will simply pass through the empty water, out the other side, un-hindered.
While the amount of cloudiness (or turbidity) of the beam could give you a measurable amount of particles for this visual indication, it's to teach you that even though your Lab PPM/TDS meters aren't reading true particulate PPMS, or not many.

### PWT Meters

The more expensive and much harder to come by meter is the PWT meter which is more accurate and only read 0-99 ppm using u/S (microseimens) and not standard TDS (total dissolved solids) and is fairl;y useful for measuring the elusive Nanoparticles. It is still not as efficient or accurate as outside lab testing and TEM (electron scanning microscope) graphics of your finished products quality.

## TYNDALL EFFECT and TESTING

Sometimes you might not have a PPM meter or you are making Colloidal solutions that the meter is NOT calibrated for, such as gold.

Unlike solutions, colloidal suspensions exhibit light scattering. A beam of light or laser, invisible in clear air or pure water, will trace a visible path through a genuine colloidal suspension, e.g. a headlight on a car shining through fog. This is known as the Tyndall effect (after its discoverer, the 19th-century British physicist John Tyndall), and is a special instance of diffraction.

This effect is often used as a measure of the existence of a colloid. It is visible in colloids as weak as 0.1 ppm (parts per million). However, there are exceptions. For example, the effect can not be seen with milk, which is a colloid. Tyndall scattering occurs when the dimensions of the particles that are causing the scattering are larger than the wavelength of the radiation that is scattered. It is caused by reflection of the incident radiation from the surfaces of the particles, reflection from the interior walls of the particles, and refraction and diffraction of the radiation as it passes through the particles.

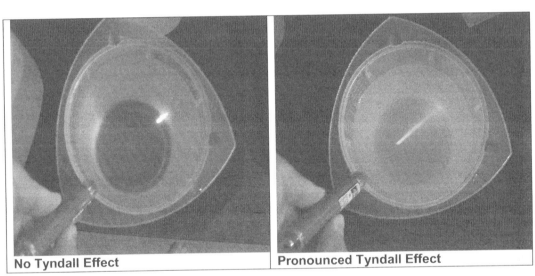

| No Tyndall Effect | Pronounced Tyndall Effect |

## WHEN USING HVAC - TESTING YOUR PPM LEVELS - GROUND OUT THE BATCH ELECTRODES

Once you turn **off** the power, it is **always IMPERATIVE to SHORT OUT or GROUND** the Anode tip INTO the water against the cathode tip, so that any stray voltage won't shock you and instead will bleed off into the batch. NST and HVAC power supplies can remain charged for up to 5 minutes when left alone and not grounded out properly.

### TO GROUND OUT or BLEED OFF that remaining CHARGE

Just disconnect both lead sets (red and black) from the gold electrode or tsm electrode tips or holders. Re-adjust your electrodes to desired depths and distance, re-hook up the alligator clips and lead sets and power back up to see result. Be careful, the TIP of the ANODE ELECTRODE MAY BE RED HOT, you can get burned, use your non-conductive tool to do this safely!

*TESTING NOTE: Always use the full GROUND OUT procedure above or at least wait a couple of minutes BEFORE DIPPING YOUR PPM METER INTO A BREWING BATCH or use the quicker GROUNDING METHOD as mentioned above, before TESTING your batch with your PPM Meter, voltage onto the batch CAN RUIN YOUR PPM METER!*

## PPM METER INTERFERENCE NOTICE:

An operating and generating PS15, PS200 and NST's transmits RF energy through the air and can make sensitive PPM Meters read inaccurately, even when not dipped into a live batch. If you have odd voltages flowing around your room because of a nearby HV power supply in **OPERATION** or even in the same room as an OPERATING HV SUPPLY your PPM METER will read wildly different measurements.

We should also take a moment and alert you to the fact that if you have a **finished batch settling** nearby and have a new batch going under the PAM method on the same lab bench and you try and PPM TEST the previous settling batch, you COULD get erratic readings from the meter. WE SUGGEST THAT ALL NEARBY HV supplies are de-energized and OFF, before testing settling batches made earlier. When de-energized, dip your PPM meter into the batch and take the first reading. It will be around 0-2ppm most likely using the ARC METHOD. We suggest you turn it back on and let it run for another 15 minutes. What you are trying to do is to find out your BASE TIMELINE for your SLP Effect.

Most researchers can get their BASE TIMELINE written down after a just few experiments. They then simply set up the PAM method and let it run for the BASE TIMELINE for their particular desired PPM outcome.

If you want a higher PPM outcome or stronger batch, merely add more brewing time. You will see most QUART BATCHES take between 10-60 minutes for a small ppm reading. This may vary depending on your local SLP effect and distilled water used. If you are using ½ gallon or gallon containers, your brew time will increase exponentially.


BECAUSE OF THE PARTICULATE and NON-IONIC minerals the **PLASMA ARC METHOD** creates, your PPM meter reading will read much lower than the true batch ppm levels. The false readings in an PUAM ARC produced batch are normally about 50% or so lower than the actual, lab tested amounts.


## What is Nano-Technology?

A nanometer is one billionth of a meter; a human hair is roughly 100,000 nanometers wide. The silver nanoparticles typically measure 25nm. Nanotechnology is the ability to measure, see, manipulate and manufacture things usually between 1 and 100 nanometers. There is no accepted international definition of a nanoparticle, but one given in the new PAS71 document developed in the UK is: "A particle having one or more dimensions of the order of 100nm or less".

The Journal of Nanotechnology has published a study that found silver nanoparticles kills HIV-1 and is likely to kill virtually any other virus. The study, which was conducted by the University of Texas and Mexico University, is the first medical study to ever explore the benefits of silver nanoparticles.

Samsung Electronics released a new line of side-by-side refrigerators with advanced health-friendly features for the Korean Market. The new refrigerators are the first to use nano-silver particles in the water dispenser system and deodorizer unit. In addition, nano-technology has been applied to the vegetable compartment and "neo-fresh" compartment to create an anti-bacterial gasket. In Asia and Europe, South Korea's LG Electronics and the German unit of Daewoo already offer silver-lined refrigerators and vacuum cleaners.

Silver's antibacterial properties have been exploited in a number of applications. Western medicine has been using eye-drops containing silver to prevent infections in newborn babies' eyes for more than a century. Antibiotics such as erythromycin are now used for similar infections. Silver has also been used in salves for burn victims and to purify water.

Unlike other metals such as lead and mercury, silver is not toxic to humans and is not known to cause cancer, reproductive or neurological damage, or other chronic adverse effects. Nor has normal day-to-day contact with solid silver coins, spoons or bowls been found to affect human health.

Since ancient times, people have known of the germ-fighting qualities of silver. Dead bodies were wrapped in silver cloth to ward off bad odors. In ancient Greece and Rome, silver containers were used for perishable liquids because they retarded the growth of food-spoiling organisms.

Many apparel makers, including Adidas and Polartec, have licensed a silver-coated nylon fiber known as X-Static from Noble Biomaterials Inc. Brooks Sports introduced a line last fall touting the silver fibers' ability to promote thermal regulation as well as odor protection.

In minute concentrations, silver is highly toxic to germs while relatively non-toxic to human cells.

Silver has antibacterial, antifungal, and deodorizing effects, and has been approved by the FDA for use in beauty products.

Antibiotic drugs can be used to kill the pathogens attacked by silver nanoparticles but bacteria and viruses are becoming increasingly resistant to drug therapies. Silver nanoparticles kill all types of fungal infections, bacteria and viruses, including antibiotic resistant strains. No drug based antibiotic is effective on all types of bacteria.

## What is Hydrophasic Technology as used by Pacific-Organix?

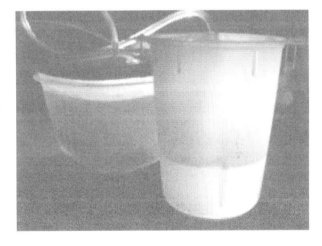

Without divulging all of our trade secrets, our Hydrophasic technology is based upon a hydrogen/oxygen splitting chamber we designed and built a few years ago in our small Portland, Oregon lab.

The Hydrophase Chamber™ as we have licensed it today, take regular distilled water and creates structured water with split hydrogen and oxygen molecule. While it is split, the molecules are excited by high voltage and each are charged electrostatically with a proper ion.

When brought back together, the distilled water has a structural bond of close to 114° instead of the stand 100-104° bonding.

The batch of water comes out of the Hydrophasic Chamber more purified and structurally bonded with the aide effect of the batch becomes saturated and infused with hyper-oxygen.

In fact, before we treat the batch, it can be literally used to fire plasma cutters, and flames, because its by-product is a mild form of hydrogen liquefied water.

This new technology, when added to our Nano-Technology creates the most bio-efficient colloidal product that has been independently lab tested on Earth today. If you want to try some out, please visit our retail site at www.pacific-organix.com and look for our new 2009 Hydrophase Silver, Copper, Gold and Zinc sols.

# History of Colloidal Products, Concentrates & Topical Salves

## Colloidal Silver A Booket

Colloidal silver appears to be a powerful, natural antibiotic and preventative against infections. Acting as a catalyst, it reportedly disables the enzyme that one-celled bacteria, viruses and fungi need for their oxygen metabolism. They suffocate without corresponding harm occurring to human enzymes or parts of the human body chemistry. The result is the destruction of disease-causing organisms in the body and in the food.

## Early Research

Colloidal silver was in common use until 1938. Many remember their grandparents putting silver dollars in milk to prolong its freshness at room temperature. At the turn of the century, scientists had discovered that the body's most important fluids are colloidal in nature: suspended ultra-fine particles. Blood, for example, carries nutrition and oxygen to the body cells.

This led to studies with colloidal silver. Prior to 1938, colloidal silver was used by physicians as a mainstream antibiotic treatment and was considered quite "high-tech." Production methods, however, were costly. The pharmaceutical industry moved in, causing colloidal research to be set aside in favor of fast working and financially lucrative drugs.

The Food and Drug Administration today classifies colloidal silver as a pre-1938 drug. A letter from the FDA dated 9/13/91 states: "These products may continue to be marketed as long as they are advertised and labeled for the same use as in 1938 and as long as they are manufactured in the original manner."

Some of the manufacturing methods used before 1938 are still used today. An electro-colloidal process, which is known to be the best method, is used.
Contemporary Studies

While studying regeneration of limbs, spinal cords and organs in the late 1970s, Robert O. Becker, M.D., author of The Body Electric, discovered that silver ions promote bone growth and kill surrounding bacteria. The March 1978 issue of Science Digest, in an article, "Our Mightiest Germ Fighter," reported: "Thanks to eye-opening research, silver is emerging as a wonder of modern medicine. An antibiotic kills perhaps a half-dozen different disease organisms, but silver kills some 650 pathogens, not actual diseases.

Resistant strains fail to develop. Moreover, silver is virtually non-toxic." The article ended with a quote by Dr. Harry Margraf, a biochemist and pioneering silver researcher who worked with the late Carl Moyer, M.D., chairman of Washington University's Department of Surgery in the 1970s: "Silver is the best all-around germ fighter we have."

## How It Works

The presence of colloidal silver near a virus, fungus, bacterium or any other single celled pathogen disables its oxygen metabolism enzyme, its chemical lung, so to say. Within a few minutes, the pathogen suffocates and dies, and is cleared out of the body by the immune, lymphatic and elimination systems. Unlike pharmaceutical antibiotics, which destroy beneficial enzymes, colloidal silver leaves these tissue-cell enzymes intact, as they are radically different from the enzymes of primitive single-celled life.

Thus (properly produced) colloidal silver is absolutely safe for humans, reptiles, plants and all multi-celled living matter.

## Product Quality

Many brands of colloidal silver are inferior. The highest grade is produced by the electro-colloidal non-chemical method where the silver particles and water have been colloided, i.e., dispersed within and bound to each other by an electric current. The super-fine silver particles are suspended indefinitely in distilled water.

The ideal color of colloidal silver is a clear to golden yellow. Darker colors indicate larger silver particles that tend to collect at the bottom of the container and are not true colloids. If a product contains a stabilizer or lists trace elements other than silver, or if it needs to be shaken, it is inferior. If a product requires refrigeration, some other ingredient is present that could spoil.

The container and dropper must be glass, as plastic cannot preserve the silver in liquid suspension for any length of time. Some brands with high concentrations of silver may actually not be completely safe. High concentrations of silver do not kill disease germs more effectively than the safe range of 3 to 5 parts per million (ppm.).

## Ingesting Colloidal Silver

Taken orally, the silver solution is absorbed from the mouth into the bloodstream, then transported quickly to the body cells. Swishing the solution under the tongue briefly before swallowing may result in faster absorption. In three to four days the silver may accumulate in the tissues sufficiently for benefits to begin. Colloidal silver is eliminated by the kidneys, lymph system and bowel after several weeks.

If routinely exposed to dangerous pathogenic germs, some recommend a regular daily intake as a protection. In cases of minor burns, an accumulation of colloidal silver may hasten healing, reducing the possibility of scar tissue and infection. It is believed by many in the natural healing arts that the lives of millions of people who are susceptible to chronic low-grade infections can be enhanced by this preventative health measure.
Chronic or Serious Conditions

1 teaspoon of 5 ppm. colloidal silver equals about 25 micrograms (mcg.) of silver. 1 - 4 teaspoons per day (25 - 100 mcg.) is generally considered to be a "nutritional amount" and is reported to be safe to use for extended periods of time. Amounts higher than this are generally considered "therapeutic amounts" and should only be used periodically.

In cases of illness, natural health practitioners have often recommended taking double or triple the "nutritional amount" for 30 to 45 days, then dropping down to a smaller maintenance dose.

Amounts from 1 - 32 ounces per day have reportedly been used in acute conditions.  If your body is extremely ill or toxic, do not be in a hurry to clear up everything at once. If pathogens are killed off too quickly, the body's five eliminatory channels (liver, kidneys, skin, lungs and bowel) may be temporarily overloaded, causing flu-like conditions, headache, extreme fatigue, dizziness, nausea or aching muscles.

Ease off on the colloidal silver to a smaller amount and increase your distilled water intake. Regular bowel movements are a must in order to relieve the discomforts of detoxification. Resolve to reduce sugar and saturated fats from the diet, and exercise more. Given the opportunity, the body's natural ability to heal may amaze you.

### Topical Uses

Some have used colloidal silver in a nasal spray mister - to reach the sinuses and nasal passages.

Spray bottles have been used for topical use on kitchen and bathroom surfaces, skin, sore throat, eyes, burns, etc. Colloidal silver is painless on cuts, abrasions, in open wounds, in the nostrils for a stuffy nose, and even in a baby's eyes because, unlike some antiseptics, it does not destroy tissue cells. It's excellent as an underarm deodorant, since most underarm odor is caused by bacteria breaking down substances released by the sweat glands!

### Colloidal Concentrates

Let your batches brew to about 30-100ppm (Silver) this batch make look dark yellow or gray colored, decant, or filter and then add it to any of the Herbal Topical Cream recipes below. Don't INGEST Colloidal Concentrates.

### Some Common Uses of Colloidal Silver

Natural health practitioners have for years recommended taking one tablespoon daily, for four days, to establish a level, then one teaspoon daily for maintenance (proportional to body weight for children). After six weeks, a pause of several weeks has also been recommended by some natural healing arts doctors. Also, colloidal silver can be applied directly to cuts, scrapes, and open sores, or on a bandage for warts. It can be applied on eczema, itches, acne or bug bites. To purify water, add one tablespoon per gallon, shake well and wait six minutes. Mixed this way, it's tasteless. It is not an allopathic poison.

### Veterinary and Garden Use

Colloidal silver has worked just as well on pets of all kinds. Used in proportion to body weight, it should bring the same results. In the garden, field or greenhouse, add enough to the water or soil - and the plants will do the rest.

### Tolerance To Disease Organisms

We have all heard of the "super-germs" that are resistant to most modern antibiotics. Some believe that single-celled germs cannot mutate into silver-resistant forms, as happens with conventional antibiotics.

Therefore no tolerance to colloidal silver would develop through mutation. Also, colloidal silver has not been demonstrated to interact or interfere with other medicines being taken. Inside the body, silver apparently does not form toxic compounds or react with anything other than a germ's oxygen-metabolizing enzyme. Colloidal silver may truly be a safe, natural remedy for many of mankind's ills. Additionally, there has never been a drug interaction reported between colloidal silver and any other medication. It's difficult to overdose - unless large amounts are ingested. Colloidal silver has been reported by users to be both a remedy and prevention for numerous infections, colds, flus, and fermentations due to various bacteria, viruses or fungi, even the non-apparent low-grade, general body infections many people have.

Living organisms are in the colloidal chemical state, not the crystalline state. Substances already in that form may be more readily assimilated by the body. Colloidal silver is the most useable form of a reputedly effective germ fighter.

A colloidal suspension is ultra-fine particles of one substance, suspended by an electric charge in another substance. Homogenized milk and aerosol sprays are colloidal suspensions. Colloidal silver is pure, metallic silver (not a chemical compound) of particles 15 atoms or fewer, each with a positive electric charge, and attached to a molecule of simple protein. This new particle floats in pure water. The electric charge is stronger than gravity so the silver particles don't sink.

## Colloidal Silver in Advance of Illness?

When the possibility of germ exposure is higher, colloidal silver can be taken orally each day or applied topically when there is a skin problem. It's like having a second defense system. The silver acts only as a catalyst and is stabilized. It is non-toxic, except to one-cell plants and animals, and is non-addicting. It also apparently kills parasites because they have a one cell egg stage in their reproductive cycle.

Older folks reportedly feel younger because their body energies are used for other uses than constantly fighting disease. Digestion has also been reportedly better. Medical research has shown that silver promotes more rapid healing, with less scar tissue, even in the case of severe burns.

Successes have been reported in cases that previously have been given up by established doctors. Colloidal silver is tasteless and won't sting even a baby's eyes, and won't upset your stomach.

As stated earlier, if you do ingest a daily dose of colloidal silver, you should do it in small amounts, not exceeding the recommended daily dose of 2 tablespoons twice daily for an adult or half of that for a child.

Also take a Probiotic to help combat the silvers wide bacteria killing properties as before mentioned. Killing off your good intestinal flora weakens your immune system faster than any flu or cold virus.

When ingesting any colloidal product, it is a well known fact to swish the liquid around for 30 seconds before swallowing it. This will make any of the colloidal mineral liquids much more efficient.

Please do not use any colloidal products made in a non-sterile, non-FDA registered lab for intravenous use, as it has not been properly filtered. Such IV use of colloidal silver is unwise as it could actual cause staph infections, vein collapse after prolonged use and other skin problems.

I have so many clients and field producers who have life threatening diseases like HIV that want to use these product via IV methods and it is our recommendation that you do not attempt to use it as such.

To bring a colloidal mineral into USP grade, you would need to sterilize it and micron filter it to the point that it would trap almost 70% of all the pathogen fighting particles. I have yet to see any blood work or lab results showing a significant decrease in HIV virus over just ingesting it orally. Remember, you already own the most effective blood filter known to man, it is your liver.

There are recent (non-scientific) studies and comparisons of my clients blood/lab results that actually showed that by using the newer Nano-Silver in the above 10ppm strength (18 ppm was the best targeted range) that the HIV Viral loads remained constant ot the same while on a 3 and 6 month trial of potent NanoSilver, however, each individual case was finally required to go onto HAART meds, because it appeared from our non-scientific case studies, that the NanoSilver was only able to slow the progression of the HIV replication to a certain point and then became ineffective in each case.

The final result was interesting as it was assumed that NanoSilver cannot be used so much as to build up a bodies immune response and make it unusable. However, it appears that the HIV virus actually found a way to replicate once again, in with high levels of NanoSilver trying to suppress the virus inside the body.

The comparison study concluded that NanoSilver and other colloidal therapy products only slow or temporarily stopped the virus. It could not kill or other suffocate the virus as earlier University Studies suggested in the 1990's. The point is, if your client or even yourself has HIV, there is currently no alternative therapy that can honestly cure or treat the disease as of this report, 2008.

## Colloidal Silver Overdose

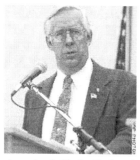

It is so important for researchers, producers and customers to realize that too much of any one thing is bad. This includes improperly made colloidal silver.

While we have no reports of toxification from Colloidal Zinc, Copper and Gold; Colloidal Silver, when IMPROPERLY MADE and ingested can cause a permanent skin discoloration called ARGRIA.

Argyria is a dermatological condition in which the skin changes in pigment from its natural color to a grayish-blue. The condition occurs as a result of cumulative exposure to silver nitrates or silver salts, which over time percolate into the dermis. Initially tinting it a pallid bluebell, continued treatment tarnishes the skin first to slate, then puce, then finally a dull confederate grey. This is made worse by going into the sun, tanning and for those that have to work outside. There have never been any reports of PROPERLY MADE SILVER causing Argyria, because we teach you to produce Colloidal Silver with only electrical energy, pure distilled water and clean lab supplies. ALL of the Argyria sufferers have gone on record to state they made their own super high ppm, yellow to gray colloidal silver, by using table salts to make silver nitrate or chlorides. Adding salt makes any colloidal process happen at about 1000 times the rate of normal, natural colloidal dispersion we teach.

After ingestion, silver salts are deposited in the skin and **oxidized by sunlight**, via the same process that develops photographs. Discoloration is first noticeable in the fingernails; gradually it spreads to the face and gums, and eventually the whole body. Face creams containing silver can even result in a bluish-brown discoloration of the eyeballs themselves. While Argyria has no real side effects aside from a slight itching, the condition is irreversible since silver becomes trapped in the deepest layers of skin. Some sufferers have tried "dermabrading", a painful-sounding surgical process which strips the top layers of skin from the face, though little success has been shown.

Most people afflicted with Argyria -- or its sister disease, Chrysiasis (discoloration due to gold overdose) -- argue that the severe social stigma associated with the disease far diminishes the benefits of the placebo effect. Sufferers find it difficult to win jobs and blowjobs while sporting the Al Jolson equivalent of AIDS spots. One need only parade across the town square with a slight list and a drool-dripping grimace to convince women and children that your sleepy town has a zombie problem. A homeless Argyria sufferer asleep on a park bench might be awakened by paramedics trying CPR, afraid that the local wino has stopped breathing. A hundred years ago, syphilitic Argyria sufferers pranced about circus sideshows as the Incredible Blue Man; nowadays a few of these lazars find work as mimes doing the robot at tourist hotspots, but nobody's buying it.

 Starting in 1999, Montana native Stan Jones (pictured above) drank up to 16 full ounces of overkill 100-500 ppm of colloidal silver he made using 9 volt, unregulated batteries and table salt. He believed it to be a natural antibiotic which would save him from the forecasted Y2K disaster, with its exploding toilets, scant antibiotics, and menacing clouds of anthrax. Jones would later emerge transformed from his sun-dappled home on the Gallatin River, entering the 2002 Montana senate race as the first blue Libertarian candidate.

Soon Jones was making Oddly Enough... headlines across the country, as both a colloidal silver sufferer and a supporter of the practice. Citing his recent lack of colds and other maladies, he became the first high-profile pusher of the alternative medicine in decades, despite his complexion: "It's my fault that I overdosed, but I still believe it's the best antibiotic in the world," Jones said.

## Pushing your Batch Limits

We are always in contact with our Scientific and Research Customers who report back that our standards and limits of 10 ppm (clear colored) ranges for LVDC –Ionic made silver is more than safe.

### 2008 Ionic Silver Bio-Efficiency tests:

We have learned that several accredited labs have been working on in vitro bio efficiency tests in 2008. They tested various types of colloidal silver at different strengths on viruses in a lab petri dish. They shared some data we are allowed to publish here and we were told that for LVDC – Ionic silver, the silver did not significantly kill the virus until it reached 15-18 ppm or over. Of course, the by-product of this 18 ppm ionic batch was that its color range was dark golden or grey colored and had showed signs of particle conglomeration and batch saturation. To most producers, this would be a ruined batch, only good for topical use.

### 2008 HVAC Nano Silver Bio-Efficiency tests:

A similar test was accomplished on HVAC produced particulate silver and the ppm amount needed to kill the same test virus was between 12-15 ppm. To reach this ppm amount, the lab was required to brew a 1000ml batch of particulate silver for almost 12 hours. So there are trade-offs in producing each product to meet the labs bio-efficiency target point.

### So, how can we meet the target and still stay within the limitations of the batch?

With Ionic batches, one way is to add a few drops of H2O2 and increase the electrode wetted depth or double the silver electrode density (bigger electrode plates). Also using electrode swapping techniques and wiping down the electrodes several times through a batch, once can conceive of pushing an ionic batch to 18 ppm and still maintain the crystal clear color. Also, reducing the batch current to under 5 ma on the electrodes and reducing voltage from 30 vdc to 15 may slow the process down enough to slowly push a batch past its saturation point and into the ppm ranges needed.

With particulate batches, one can also add a few drops of H2O2 as well and increase the electrode wetted surface area by using silver plates instead of silver wire electrodes.

Both batches need to be brewed using constant aeration or stirring and both batches will require a significant brew time increase from 4 to 8 hours. Keeping the batch container small will also help increase the batch progression. Using larger brew containers makes the process less controllable.

The lab suggests trying different distilled water brands as well as trying experiments with DEIONISED water to help push the batch to the target area.

Unfortunately, this has been a producers problem for years, just how to make the highest ppm batch, while maintaining the smallest particle for the best bio-efficiency.

Some labs are trying to make the conglomerated 18-20 ppm bathes and then micron filtering them to catch the big particle, however, they see their ppm count drop in the end and have been unable to certify their products efficiency.

# Using the PUAM Method for making Industrial Strength Nano Silver, Zinc and Copper

PLASMA UNDERWATER ARC METHOD
GLASS BATCH CONTAINER

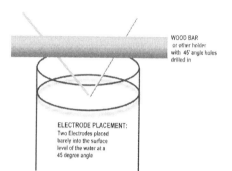

WOOD BAR
or other holder
with 45' angle holes
drilled in

ELECTRODE PLACEMENT:
Two Electrodes placed
barely into the surface
level of the water at a
45 degree angle

Besides the slower (and more controlled) TSM brewing method for HVAC Silver, Copper and Zinc, we have tested using the PUAM (shown left) for other phases of Colloidal production.

Once only thought to have been beneficial in PUAM Gold production, we have learned that you can Arc or 'sputter' electrode tip ends of various colloidal metals, such as silver, copper and zinc.

Of course the downside of any PUAM method where the electrodes come into nanosecond contact with each other, thousands of times per hour, is that your electrodes wear down very rapidly.

Also, we have learned that the particle size increases from the normal 10-30 nm size to charged particulates of 100-500 nanometer size. This is great news for topical uses and possibly as additives to Pools and Spas, and the particle stay mostly (about 90%) in phase and suspended in the liquid they were brewed in.

It is recommended that producers wishing to experiment with the PUAM methods to achieve a HIGHER PPM batch outcome, without additives, use this method. It is also recommended that you use a 60ma or 120 ma NST or advanced power supply. Voltages can be as little as 7.5 KV all the way up to 15 kv.

Using the PUAM to make silver, causes the batch to rapidly turn light yellow and then darker yellow. This is indicative of the larger 300-500 nm size particles you are creating.

The brew time averages about 90 minutes for a 1000 ml beaker at abo0ut 15-20 ppm outcome (m/s ppm) all without additives, H2O2 or booster chemicals. Using the PUAM method requires CONSTANT ADJUSTMENT of the electrode tips to keep the arc or the 'smoking tips' working with any efficiency.

Do not let the tip ends 'weld' or stick together for very long, as this can damage your power supply. Using your DIGIPRO power supply to make these other minerals or to push a batch past 10 ppm is not advisable and you assume all risks for safety and damage to yourself or your equipment.

We recommended that you NOT use any additives at all, but field researchers are reporting they are able to push a batch farther than 10 ppm when using salines, H2O2 or other additives.

Here are our results with trying to 'push' a 1000 ml batch to 20 ppm or higher without any additive, just simple distilled water as the base that was rated at 1 ppm pre base line testing.

| Mineral | PPM | Color | Brew Time |
|---|---|---|---|
| NanoSilver | 15-20 | light yellow | 90 minutes |
| NanoCopper | 18-22 | light yellow | 80 minutes |
| NanoZinc | 16-20 | light clear/blue | 90 minutes |

# HVAC – QPC SETUP
### For the DIGIPRO NST, PS1500, PS2000 High Voltage systems
### ADDENDEUM – 2008 Version 3

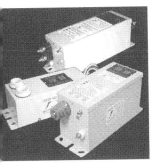

## Special Set-Up Instructions
## *EXTREME DANGER*
*HIGH VOLTAGE OUTPUT CAN KILL YOU SO USE AT YOUR OWN RISK! You must be trained to use this item!*

NST (Neon Sign Transformer) KIT comes unassembled and you are required to installed power cords and HV lead set and clips to make it fully functional. Some models have Auto Regulation Circuitry and Ground Fault UL listed models meet or exceed UL 2161. Please do not disable these devices.

**Model: DIGIPRO NST 15 KV at 30ma max**
**DO NOT SHORT OUT LEADS OR ALLIGATOR CLIPS UNINTENTIONALLY**
**Do not disable the Ground Fault Safety System**

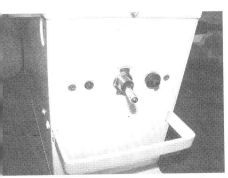

**Refer to Picture (left)**
Your DIGIPRO NST will look similar to this unit pictured left. On the control panel, you will see (starting from left to right) a red LED light, this is your computerized diagnostic light. The light steady, blinking or 'off' states are listed on the back Caution/LED label.

In the middle of your NST, you will find a standard toggle switch or a switch that may look like a standard home light switch. This is the **main power switch** and turns ON and OFF the power of the power supply. When turned 'ON' the red LED light should come on and remain on steadily throughout your production batches. The right (small) pushbutton is for resetting your NST's computer mode, or for use in forcing it into a 30 minute timed 'by-pass' mode.

**DO NOT USE THE BY-PASS** mode for regular colloidal production, it is usually never necessary as the standard 'smart mode' will work for single, up through 4 batch loads. The by-pass mode is for advanced testing and to trouble shoot your NST should it get shorted out and need to be reset. The instructions about this Mode switch are included on the side label as well as the included NST manufacture addendums. The Computer LED diagnostics and the troubleshooting push button and provided as a safe guard against damaging your power supply. Things that can reset or cause the power supply to go into troubleshoot mode (or events where you need to troubleshoot) are usually accidentally shorting out the electrodes, leadsets or other accidental or unintended shorts, last for more than 30 seconds, overheating or lastly, NST coil damage.

As of March, 2008, Pride Labs has over fifty NST and fifteen PS1500's running in customers labs and homes. Pride Labs does not build or fix the NST units and the customer is required to return it directory to the manufacture if a unit goes out. With that being said, as of March 2008, we have never seen a single NST or PS-1500 returned for repair, nor have any customers had to send their NST back directly to the factory while under the power supplies factory 1 year warranty. We believe this is due to customer following our methods and experiments to the letter and not by deviating from our tested and proven experiments.
The DIGIPRO NST has an automatically adjusting Voltage and Current computer board housed in the front chamber of the power supplies box, this constantly samples the HVAC output and feedback current or load of your batches. Using one batch at a time is the 'norm' while users can chain up to four QPC-32's (or other beaker) batches simultaneously for the normal TSM method of production, as discussed and

taught in our Colloidal Production Book, that should have been included when you purchased your kit. There is a downside to chaining multiple TSM batches, as the NST (and your batches can heat up) this is normal, but to stay on the safe side, we suggest NEVER RUNNING YOUR NST or PS-15000 HVAC experiment longer than 2 hours, with an hour of cool-down in between experiments. Most experiments only require about 60-90 min max anyway.

This computer board also acts as a second generation, Fully UL listed separate ground fault device that *might help ramp down the voltage and current if you get shocked. Of course you will NOT EVER GET SHOCKED if you remember to TURN OFF the main toggle switch AND or install the power supply on a power strip with a lighted ON/OFF switch. You will also NEVER get shocked if you DO NOT ADJUST any electrodes, leadsets or alligator clips, QPC-32 containers or batches WHILE THE POWER IS ON!

**POWER SWITCH:** Your NST should have come with a POWER ON/OFF toggle Switch built onto the side of the NST Box (not included in 220-277 International Models). If your NST does not have an ON/OFF toggle switch, you will need to provide a GROUNDED POWER STRIP with on/off switch to power on and off your NST Unit.

**We suggest that you buy a SURGE PROECTED GFII style power strip to add an extra layer of SHOCK PROTECTION.**


## POWER LEADS/LEADSET

Your included HV main cables coming out of the power supply are rated for 15KV or more (your system will never actually put out that much into a colloidal batch) it actually only puts out a few thousand volts and about 2 to 3 ma of current into your given colloidal batch, but this can still zap your hands.

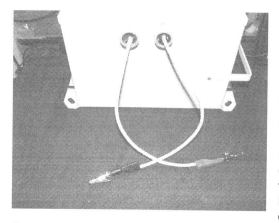

Being an electronic technician, I have been zapped by brushing my hand against an active Nano Silver batch and I really felt it, but in comparison to regular home 120 vac house current, it was VERY minor and caused no burning or muscle contraction like the many times I have been shocked by household current. You see, your home ac power is low voltage but SUPER high current (over 100 amps) so the current is what gets you!

Included on the main white HV leads, is 50 KV alligator clamps. Please do not let them touch UNINTENTIONALLY while the NST is powered ON. The Clips are marked RED/BLACK, however, with HVAC processes, the electrodes polarity swap from negative to positive 50-60 times per minute.

**About Lead sets, Clamps, Shocks, Sparking and Sizzles**

When working with HVAC experiments, try to keep all your leadset wires from touching or even crossing over each other as they COULD arc or quietly drain off precious HVAC voltage the electrodes down in your beakers or QPC's need.

**If you see sparks, arcs or hear sizzling sounds**, take a look at your leadset positions and move them or spread them farther apart. Again, please don't adjust leadsets, alligator clip or cables WHILE your power supply is on. You can use a wooden spoon, glass tube or plastic item to remotely adjust leadsets and clamps WHILE the unit is on, just remember to keep you hand 6 to 10" away at all times. This means your non-metallic tool needs to be about 12" in length. Make sure your tool isn't wet, moist or soggy, water acts as a great path along the tool to zap you.

Make sure your NST is NOT set up on a Metal Bench, metal work table or other metal surface as it is possible small arcs CAN literally pop out of weak points along even brand new leadsets. Leadset plastic covering and coatings are rated to protect the user against many thousands of volts, BUT I would NEVER dare to brush up against them, even accidentally, while I have a batch going.

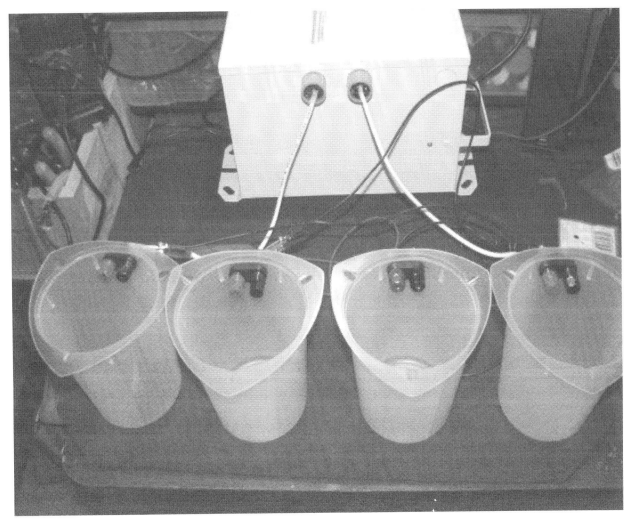

### Setting up chained batches and the QPC-32 beaker system
You **MUST** setup your NST unit in a clear and open bench, table or lab area to be able to SAFELY chain multiple HVAC batches. The setup in the **picture left** shows an NST with four QPC-32's lined up.

We suggest that you spread out your batches and beakers farther than what the picture depicts. By placing the beakers 4-6" apart from each other, you will be able to more accurately adjust and stir the batches while they are being made and your individual leadsets will not get so crossed with each other.

Chaining multiple batches is how you will really learn about stray voltage, arcs, sparks and sizzles, because if you cross two many reds over black lines, you may get a short (even through the wires insulation) that could damage the leadsets. This is the beast called HVAC, where voltages can fly out like baby pieces of lightening, searching for the least resistance to ground OR the other set.

Your kit may have included a SECONDARY SET of lead sets (usually red and black) cables and they all have pre-installed STACKABLE ALLIGATOR CLAMPS or jacks. They slide into each other as depicted in the series of photos below:

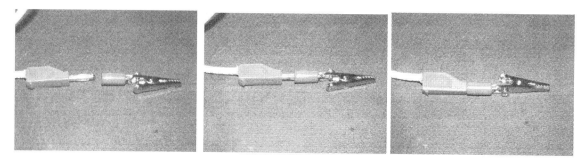

Placing the white rubber HV cable (plug) into the back of the Industry standard alligator clips

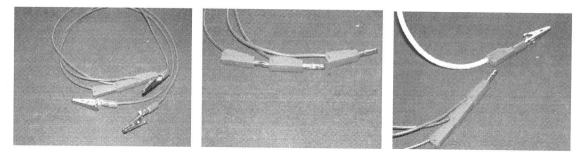

Pre-stacked secondary batch leadsets plugs slide into back hole (port) on each other
Lastly, the secondary red/black leadsets are all stacked and can be slid into the main or mater alligator jack)

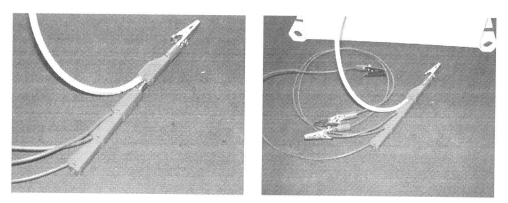

The secondary red/black leadsets are plugged into the Master /Primary white leadset coming out of the NST or PS-2000 ports. The pic above shows how the 3 secondary leadsets fit into the master/primary rear stacking port. You have finished with the red set, not duplicate the past 6 pictures with the black primary and secondary leads.

# QPC SET UP

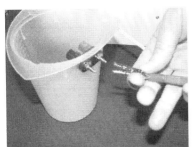 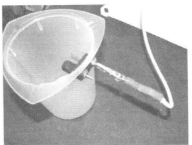 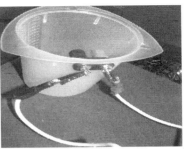

**If you are going to do a single batch, just clip the alligator camp onto the QPC-32 rear electrode holding terminal as shown. You can do this straight on or for further safety and less chance of alligator clip to alligator arcing, your can set your clamps as shown in the pic on the right.**

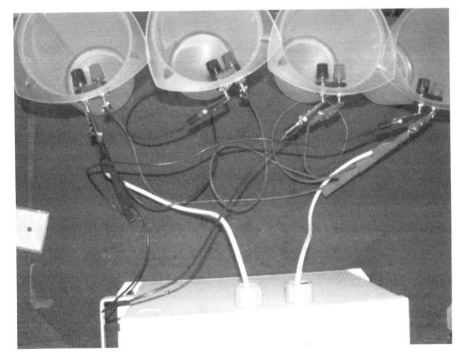

## TO AVOID ARCING:

When using two or more batch containers simultaneously, please try to separate the primary and secondary leadsets as much as possible.

It **IS OK** to cross red with red and black with black,

It **IS NOT OK** to cross red with black!

Try to keep the red and black leads separate by a couple inches if possible.

## ELECTRODE ADJUSTMENT UNDER FULL POWER:

Please DO NOT adjust your electrodes while the NST Power is going and the lead sets are connected to the electrodes. You can be SHOCKED and KILLED by attempting to adjust an experiment (especially underwater arc gold) under any HV power.

**Always turn off your power supply and wait 15 seconds for it to DISCHARGE before attempting any ELECTRODE adjustment.**

**FREE HELP 24/7 Email us** mfp.pacific@gmail.com

Here is a compilation of older, outdated experiments. These were thought at the time to be the best colloidal production experiments at the time, however, lab testing and client results proved otherwise.

They are being reproduced so that you, the field colloidal researcher, can get ideas from these experiments and possibly help you to create your own new, state of the art production methods.

## OUTDATED PAM METHOD – FOR INFORMATIONAL USE ONLY

### POAAM ™ (Plasma Open Air Arc Method)

This experiment creates fast colloidal products; however it has several PROS and CONS.

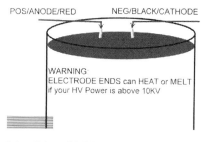

DUAL PLASMA ARC METHOD

POS/ANODE/RED    NEG/BLACK/CATHODE

WARNING:
ELECTRODE ENDS can HEAT or MELT
if your HV Power is above 10KV

Pros:

1- Creates fast (CLEAR ONLY) Colloidal Silver, Gold, Copper and Zinc in quart and bigger batches and in 1 to 50PPM *appx. range.

Cons:

1- Creates false PPM readings due to oxide & ozone nitric by-product build-ups. Batches need to sit, covered for 24 hours before taking a final PPM reading and then it is still only a semi accurate PPM reading.

2- Because the Arc is open air, the actual arc combines with air molecules to create ozone. While the creation of ozone is a good thing and acts as a natural air cleaner, the by-products of ozone directly above a water surface, creates tiny acid rain mist that if the ARC is powered on too HIGH, can turn into nitric acid. Nitric Acid can make your batches taste metallic and acidic.

The PH changes due to this effect and can actually be tough on a stomach.

3- To minimize Ozone and Acidic build-up, you should be using the LOWEST power setting and the SMALLEST plasma arc as possible. Use continuous aeration and make sure your batches are not covered, that could trap even more acid mist.

Setting up the PLASMA ARC experiment is also tricky and setting the electrodes and power setting to make the arc happen safely, is tricky to say the least, but once you have got it working for the first time, subsequent setups take about 30 seconds between batches.

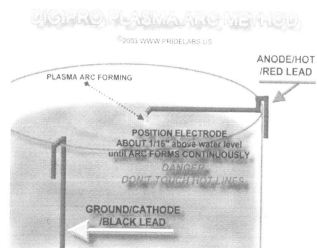

DIGIPRO PLASMA ARC METHOD

©2003 WWW.PRIDELABS.US

ANODE/HOT
/RED LEAD

PLASMA ARC FORMING

POSITION ELECTRODE
ABOUT 1/16" above water level
until ARC FORMS CONTINUOUSLY
DANGER
DON'T TOUCH HOT LINES

GROUND/CATHODE
/BLACK LEAD

Some latest research to the **Plasma Open Air Arc Method have indicated** that part of the measured (TDS/PWT) PPM readings you may receive after making a POAAM batch (up to 10-50%) you read in your batch ppm tests, are actually nitric oxide buildup or even nitric acid buildup onto the surface level of your batch. This is why we are telling all our researchers to let a PLASMA ARC BATCH set covered with a paper towel, for 24 hours, to let any nitric acid fumes bleed off.

There are ways to MINIMIZE BUILD-UPS: Some field researcher lab tests and subsequent outside lab testing show little or no oxide or acidic build-ups, but ONLY if you create your Plasma Open Air Arc methods by:

*MINIMIZING THE BREW TIME to about 15-30 minutes

*MINIMIZING your HV PLASMA ARC length (keep your arc close to the surface of the water AND use the lowest power setting to keep the minimal arc continuous).

**\*MINIMIZE your PPM FINAL RESULTS**

The PLASMA ARC creates a small lightening bolt and as a by-product causes sweet ozone air by product. While normally very healthy for air and room purification, the ozone's by-product is mostly gaseous and can turn acidic when it is brewed too long and or with too BIG of a plasma arc from tip of electrode to surface level of the batch.

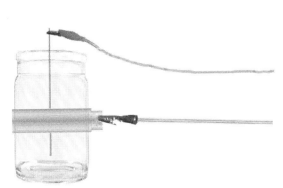

Any buildup of gaseous ozone can combine with regular air and cause a humidity problem that is close to nitric oxide buildup. This can cause toxicity concerns if you use the ARC METHOD in this fashion for longer than 30 minute periods.

We suggest stopping your PAM method at 15-30 minutes or 50 - 60 PPM (as measured on a standard PPM meter) at the maximum, to help minimize any build-up. After a 24 hour settling period, you should see the batch read about 5 to 10ppm.

## OUTDATED PAM METHOD – FOR INFORMATIONAL USE ONLY

### PTGAM (Plasma through Glass Arc Method)

This is just like the POAMM or regular PAM method talked about here in this guide with the exception that you install the ANODE electrode down into a small glass PIPETTE or test tube OR even use the SIDE of the Glass batch container, to separate the ARC from the AIR, but still touching the WATER.

This experiment that makes it impossible for any ACTUAL AIR OXIDE BUILDUPS to occur, however, without the ability to sinter off the nano-particulates via the plasma beam, like the regular PAM above accomplishes, this method may be slow and has not been tested beyond simple experimentation.

### PCM ™ (Plasma Cone Method)
Not quite the PAM (Plasma Arc Method) but pretty close to the Illustration on page three. The PCM uses the water and creates an actual vortex or 'cone' that rises up and touches the rod, even if it is hovering well above the surface of your base distilled water level.

The cone also swirls around the electrode rod at a fast pace and using a laser pen or bright spotlight flashlight, you can see the tornado effect happening. Faster then the TSM method, but about 50% slower then the advanced PCM production stated below. 20 PPM concentrations can take as long as 60 to 120 minutes or more.

## OUTDATED PAM METHOD – FOR INFORMATIONAL USE ONLY

**PGAM (Plasma Glass Arc Method)**
**This method is made up of several experiments, see illustrations below:**

The PGAM experiment uses your SIDE of your glass container, to form the PLASMA ARC through the glass, down into the BATCH LIQUID. This creates A LOT OF OZONE, which is beneficial to healthy rooms. This OZANE (when used with the older Plasma Arc Method) can cause gaseous buildup in prolonged batch sessions.

So we came up with this experiment, that DOES NOT allow the actual plasma Arc to form via AIR, but rather through the thin glass wall of your BATCH CONTAINER. This EXPERIMENT must be used with

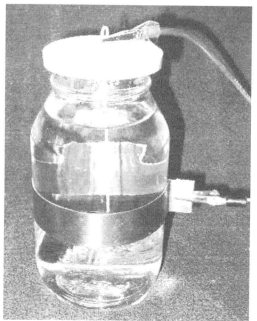

THINWALL Glass, BOMEX or LAB BEAKERS, some MASON Jars are too thick, but they will work, just much slower.

**DO NOT USE ANY PLASTIC BATCH CONTAINERS, you will MELT THEM!**
The ANODE (outside the container) electrode should be attached at the LIP of the batch container as usual, just reversed, because we are using the OUTSIDE of the glass batch container, instead of the inside this time.

Bend the ANODE as seen on the left picture, place the END or TIP of the ANODE ELECTRODE down about 1" BELOW the surface level of the inside water. This will enable the plasma arc to actually go into the water and NOT the other electrode or any AIR.

THE PLASMA ARC that will form can SHOCK YOU, be careful! We suggest you START THE ARC about 25% up on the VOLTAGE LEVEL CONTROL and then decrease the output down until the ARC almost disappears.

We do NOT SUGGEST YOU TURN IT UP FULL, although it will speed up the process, the arc at this high of OUTPUT can cause HEATING as well as you will see a large 1 to 2" FLOWER PLASMA pattern form on the outside of your beaker.

This is really cool and pretty and pours out tons of OZONE, but it also TAXES your power supply.

**PLASMA ARC through TEST TUBE or GLASS PIPETTES** This method and illustrations to the left are for experimental use only, we have not fully explored the use of letting the ARC form through a glass tube, side wall or glass pipette, whether sealed, or unsealed, to produce results.

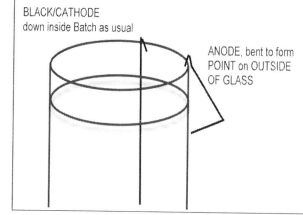

PLASMA THROUGH GLASS

GLASS BATCH CONTAINER

BLACK/CATHODE
down inside Batch as usual

ANODE, bent to form POINT on OUTSIDE OF GLASS

## OUTDATED PAM METHOD – FOR INFORMATIONAL USE ONLY

**PLASMA ARC through TEST TUBE or GLASS PIPETTES** This method and illustrations to the left are for experimental use only, we have not fully explored the use of letting the ARC form through a glass tube, side wall or glass pipette, whether sealed, or unsealed, to produce results.

### EXPERIMENT #1

This is where the anode is suspended into a regular test tube and it remains dry, you will need to push down the empty test tube into your batch about 4", we know it will try to FLOAT, we suggest you using a clothespin or clamp to hold it down into the water.

The Plasma Arc will form into the surrounded water through the glass wall of the tube.

The actual arc will not gas up and cause the amount of ozone or any possible by-products into the batch, because the arc is not physically touches the water via the air, but rather the thin glass membrane of the test tube wall.

You can also reverse this process and experiment on placing the cathode inside the pipette and let the anode produce all the particulates.

## EXPERIMENT #2
This happens when you use a glass tube or pipette that is 6" long, with the open air on each end. The electrode anode is suspended down about 5". The water is allowed to come inside and touch the anode tip inside the tube.

An alternate EXPERIMENT #2 test, is to SEAL the electrode wire at the top, so that is forms an sealed air chamber, allowing a dry air gap to be maintained from the anode tip end to the water level at the end of the pipette. Again, reversing the anode with the cathode is yet another realm of open experiments.

## OUTDATED PAM METHOD – FOR INFORMATIONAL USE ONLY

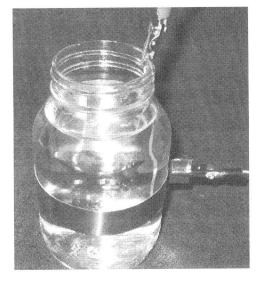

**EXPERIMENT # 3**
Required Tools:
A- PS15/PS200, PS1000 HV PLASMA ARC POWER SUPPLY
B- COPPER BAND for QUART or GALLON glass batch container

**Experiment Danger Level: MEDIUM to LOW**

Caution should be used when setting up and/or dismantling the test or while testing batches for ppm during or after the process.

Power supply should always be **off** and **discharged** fully before touching the leads, clips or container OR before trying to test the PPM of the batch using any external or handheld ppm or test meter.

## Method Advantage (OUTDATED INFO):
This experiment allows the basic PAM method to occur and make 100% nano, sub atomic particles inside the batch container DIRECTLY sintered off of the PURE ELECTROD ANODE of silver, copper, zinc or even gold. Unlike other methods that can cause odd readings and oxide levels, including acidic or nitric acid build-up, this method uses the glass batch container as a 'capacitor' to eliminate any potential oxide or by-product build-up. This process pulls solid microscopic anode particles off into the batch, leaving almost 100% PURE, particulate particles, without any IONIC properties or oxide, chloride or nitric acid buildup. The batch is also **not** ozonated to the point where the chemical process has any ability to create or add any nitric acid buildup.

# Old Style Flashlight Tyndall Line Test

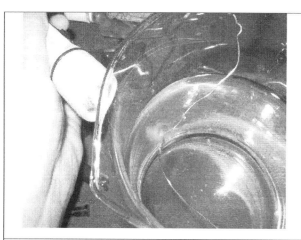

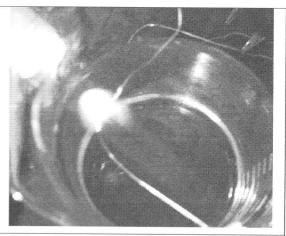

| FIG 10. UNDERWATER ARC making LVDC GOLD | FIG 11. UNDERWATER ARC making LVDC GOLD |
|---|---|
| Place the TIP of the anode right next to and almost touching the TIP of the cathode. Both tips should be under water, but near the surface. Beginning Batch, showing NO TYNDALL EFFECT | Shining a bright flashlight shows the actual particles and a good Tyndall effect. See the light beam through the water? |

## Other <u>OUTDATED</u>
## Open Air PAM Pictures

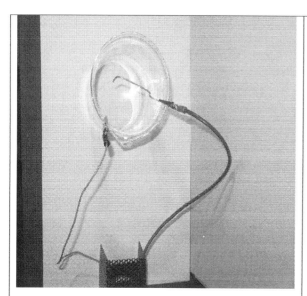

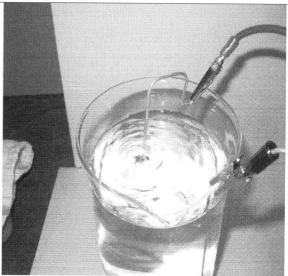

| *Top down look at a simple PAM experiment* | *Actual PAM ongoing experiment* |
|---|---|

## IDEAS FOR USING INSULATED CLAMPS (PLASTIC) TO ADJUST AN ON-GOING HV EXPERIMENT

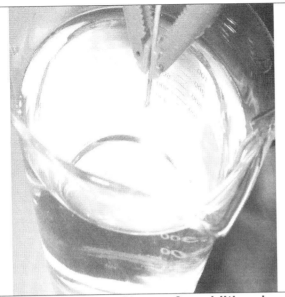

**Using Plastic Clamps for additional positions**

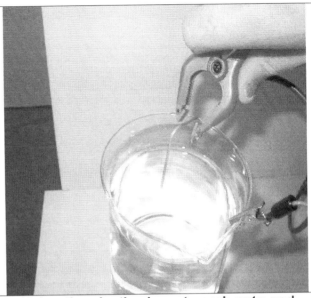

**Using the plastic clamp to grab onto and move or adjust an ongoing PAM experiment**

## ACTUAL TIMING PRODUCTION RESULT CHART
### Using Open-Air Arc (old out dated data)

| COLLOIDAL MINERAL | METHOD USED | TIME to PRODUCE 32oz | HANDHELD TDS/PPM METER FINAL READING | OUTSIDE LAB RESULT |
|---|---|---|---|---|
| Silver | PAM Open Air Arc | 35 min | 100ppm +/- 10% | 49.5 ppm +/- 10% |
| Silver | TSM | 120 min | 5 ppm +/- 10% | 9.58 ppm +/- 10% |
| Silver | PCM or TCM (cone) | 120 min | 7.5 ppm +/- 10% | 15 ppm +/- 10% |
| Copper | PAM Open Air Arc | 45 min | 120 ppm +/- 10% | 209.5 ppm +/- 10% |
| Gold | PAM Open Air Arc | 45 min | 65 ppm +/- 10% | 105 ppm +/- 10% |
| Gold | TSM | 3 hours | 5.7 ppm +/- 10% | 20.9 ppm +/- 10% |
| Gold | PCM or TCM (cone) | 3 hours | 7.1 ppm +/- 10% | 25.8 ppm +/- 10% |
| Zinc | PAM Open Air Arc | 45 min | 75.5 ppm +/- 10% | 129.0 +/- 10% |
| Zinc | TSM | 2 hours | 6 ppm +/- 10% | 15 ppm +/- 10% |

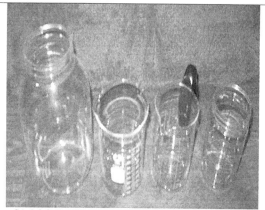

GLASS BATCH CONTAINER, YOU SUPPLY:
GALLON JAR   1000ml (34oz) Jar   32 oz Beaker/handle
32oz Jar

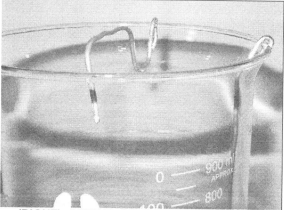

(RIGHT)  ACTUAL CATHODE (BLACK) long
Electrode placement  (LEFT) ANODE (red)
custom bent to produce PLASMA OPEN AIR ARC
ME

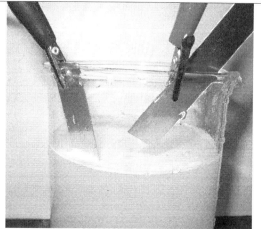

TYPICAL COPPER OR ZINC PLATE ELECTRODE
INSTALL for OPEN AIR PLASMA ARC METHOD,
cloudy water was for photo effect, not a desired
color of clear.

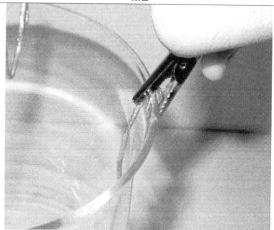

PLACE ALLIGATOR CLIP OVER THE BEND in
the ELECTRODE, both JAWS should be OVER
the inside and outside of the jar lip

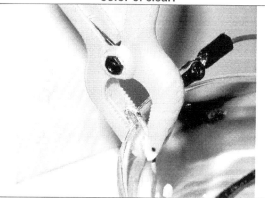

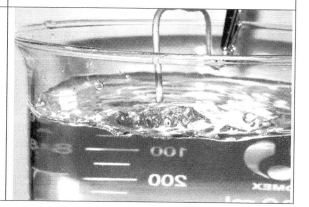

## The Metaphysics of Healing

### Ten Top Tips to Developing your Own Mental & Physical Healing Abilities

Take off your watch for at least two weeks. By doing this, you will start to gain a real sense of your own time. This is important to begin to connect with yourself, and to understand world time, universal time and how reality is shaped and created.

Make meditation a part of your life, even if it's just 10-20 minutes every other day. No need to follow complicated techniques. Just sit down and relax; be still; let your thoughts come and go; breathe deeply from the bottom of your stomach and develop awareness by being connected with yourself, the moment and all that is.

Pay attention to where you are and who you are being on a daily basis. Each day, ask yourself: Where I am right now? Who am I being? Which role am I playing? By doing this you can have more awareness of any past experience or parts of you that need healing.

Start thinking in color. When you meet someone new, ask yourself: What color are they being? Just accept the answer that comes to your mind. In time, you will develop the ability to see colors of the aura of people and objects.

Listen to yourself and your body. When you feel ill or out of balance, ask yourself why. Accept your answers. Always fulfill your needs, as unfulfilled needs create chaos.

Use Tarot cards, palmistry, astrology, crystals, runes and other means of divination at least once. These are mediums to help develop your clairvoyance (clear seeing). Don't get stuck on specific meanings; only use them as a guide. This way, you can develop your own more precise insight and gain the confidence to believe in your own thoughts and feelings.

Letting go is an important part of development. Even saying firmly in your mind twice a day: "I am letting go of everything I no longer need" will make a difference. Make time for yourself regularly. Any form a self-expression is useful, i.e. write, run, swim, play... Let yourself go in the ways that feel good to you. Remember, when you let go, you can become awake, aware and conscious.

Try a psychic development course. Remember to go at your own speed. The basics are simple. Repetition is important. Remember too that psychic abilities, healing, and awareness are already yours. You can choose to develop these abilities and use them more often.

Never compare yourself with anyone else. Realize that you too are unique and amazing. Read books, listen to tapes on the subject of development, but realize that those are guides and are for you to use as an outline to find your own ways. Be creative and listen to what you feel.

Know that anything is possible, and that nothing is ever only as it seems. Look after your body with a balanced diet and regular exercise. Each day, whenever possible, do something for your body, mind, and emotional self.


*Petrene Soames:*

*World Top Psychic, has been working with ESP and the Paranormal for over twenty years. Author of The Essence of Self-Healing (available online at timeismine.com), Petrene recognizes and values the uniqueness and individuality of each person that she encounters. "I am amazing and you are amazing too," says Petrene.*


*"Believe in yourself and let the magic be!" Visit her web site at petrene.com and enjoy her free interactive fun rooms.*

## About other herbs

So many of our clients write and want to make their own herbal and holistic medications at home, including adding colloidal products to help boost their organic made supplements, that we included several pages of organic and health related natural medicine recipes. These are included for your own personal use and we make no claim as to their worthiness as a medical herbal supplement.

Echinacea, for example, is a general immune-system enhancer often taken this way. Several species have medicinal value, but E. purpurea is one of the easiest to grow. For use in capsules, harvest and dry the above-ground portions of the plant. Taken at the first sign of a cold or flu, echinacea can be effective in boosting your immunity and relieving symptoms. The recommended dose for treating a cold is 900 milligrams a day, according to the German government's Commission E guidelines, which often are used as a standard for herbal dosages.

## Poultices:

A poultice is vegetable material, whole or mashed, which is applied externally so that the herb's properties can be absorbed by the skin. Poultices are often used to reduce inflammation, improve circulation and speed the healing of cuts, scrapes and other sores.

Comfrey, for example, has anti-inflammatory and cell-regenerating properties that can make an effective poultice for treating bruises and sprains. A comfrey poultice can be made with fresh or dry leaves — just moisten them and apply as a half-inch-thick layer, placed directly on the affected skin. Bind the poultice in place with a clean cloth.

Comfrey should not be used on deep puncture wounds because the surface can heal too quickly, trapping infection-causing bacteria inside the wound. Used externally, comfrey generally is considered safe.

## Tinctures:

A tincture is made by soaking fresh or ground herbs in alcohol to extract and preserve the active constituents of the plant. One of the advantages of tinctures is their long shelf life — most will keep for a year or longer.

Many tinctures are intended to be taken internally; often they are diluted with water and then swallowed. However, some tinctures are meant to be applied directly to the skin. For example, calendula flowers make a good first-aid tincture for treating cuts, scrapes and bruises because of the herb's antibacterial properties.

Different tincturing methods can be used, but Cech favors this approach: Begin by grinding the dried herb, or by finely mincing fresh herbs, and placing them in a quart jar. For calendula, dry the flowers and then grind them to a powder. Cover the ground or minced herbs with vodka or pure grain alcohol. If you opt for vodka, use at least 40 proof for dried herbs and 80 proof for fresh herbs; if you use pure grain alcohol, pair it with dried herbs and dilute the alcohol with distilled water at a 1-1 ratio.

Let the mixture sit, covered, for three weeks, and shake the jar daily. (Fresh herbs must remain submerged during this time because exposed plant material can rot.) After three weeks, strain the contents of the jar using a thin, clean cloth and then press the cloth to squeeze out every drop of liquid. Let the separated liquid sit overnight to settle, and then strain it again. Store the resulting herb-infused alcohol in a labeled bottle for future use.

**Infused oils:**   Some herbs have active constituents that will dissolve in vegetable oil. The resulting infused oils can be used directly by massaging them into the skin or as a base for other products such as skin creams, salves and lip balms.

Oil infused with St. John's wort, for example, is good for treating bruises, sprains, swellings, hemorrhoids and scars. Both hot- and cold-techniques can be used for infusing oils; with St. John's wort, combine one part fresh flowers and leaves by weight with three parts by volume of oil. For the hot method, place the oil and the St. John's wort in a crock pot and maintain a 110- to 120-degree temperature for two weeks. Stir daily, and at the end of the two-week period, strain the oil. For the cold method, combine the oil and herb, and then allow the mixture to sit at room temperature for at least two weeks, or until the oil has taken on the color and flavor of the leaves. Make sure the leaves remain fully submerged. Putting the infused oil in the sun will help speed the extraction process.

Although generally considered safe, St. John's wort can cause photosensitivity in some people.

### Salves and Balms:

Infused oils can be thickened into salves and balms, which many people find more convenient and less messy than the oil. Use dedicated pans and spoons to make salves and balms.

To make a salve, add two tablespoons of melted beeswax to each cup of infused oil. Melt beeswax carefully in a double boiler or over a very low flame; beeswax is flammable when overheated. (Look for beeswax online, in health food stores or from beekeepers.) Reheat the oil just enough for the wax to mix well, then let it cool. If the salve is too thick, add more oil; too thin, more wax. Oil-based salves can turn rancid over time. To help prevent this, vitamin E can be added as a preservative. In some cases, the addition of glycerin makes a smoother salve, particularly for skin creams.

All of the above preparations are called "simples" because they involve only one herb. When more than one herb is combined in such a preparation, the whole can be greater than the sum of its parts. An example of this is the Basic Balm (see recipe, Page 84); it has greater skin-toning and healing properties than a typical commercial body lotion.

For maximum effectiveness, infuse herbs individually and then combine them; more practically, infuse all the herbs for a single recipe together. Be sure to use either fresh or dried herbs; fresh herbs should be chopped or crushed before measuring.

**Teas:**  Herbal tea is another remedy made by combining multiple herbs, and most medicinal herbal teas are stronger than those sold for drinking like regular tea. To brew a medicinal tea useful for treating upset stomach, particularly as it relates to over-eating, combine equal parts of fresh or dried catnip, peppermint and chamomile. Pour a cup of boiling water over a rounded tablespoon of the herbs and let them steep for at least 15 minutes. Strain, if necessary, and drink, hot or cold. Alternatively, using do-it-yourself tea bags will eliminate the need to strain the tea.

### Basic Balm

*3 cups olive oil*
*10 tablespoons comfrey leaves*
*10 tablespoons calendula flowers*
*8 tablespoons lavender flowers*
*5 tablespoons plantain*
*5 tablespoons yarrow flowers*
*4 tablespoons sage*
*4 tablespoons beeswax granules*
*1 ounce vitamin E oil*

Infuse the herbs in the oil. Measure the infused oil and add additional oil to make 2 cups. Add the beeswax and heat; remove from the heat as soon as the wax melts and stir gently until the balm starts to thicken. Add the glycerin and stir until the mix is cool and creamy. Stir in the vitamin E oil. The balm will thicken more overnight. Generally considered safe for external use, but sage may irritate sensitive skin.

## A LITTLE BEEWAX INFO

Beeswax is a byproduct of honey production. It makes wonderful lip balms, hand lotions, hand creams, moisturizers, in cosmetics, wood finishes, waxes, leather polishes; waterproofing products, and dental molds.

It is impervious to water and unaffected by mildew. It has a melting point of 143 to 148 degrees F. and should only be heated using a double boiler as it is flammable when subjected to fire and flames. It is pliable at 100 degrees F. Beeswax is produced by the (female) worker honeybees. The wax is secreted from wax glands on the underside of the bee's abdomen and is molded into six-sided cells which are filled with honey, then capped with more wax. When honey is harvested, the top layer of wax that covers the cells, the cappings, must be removed from each hexagon shaped cell.

Bees use their wax to "glue" together the wooden frames in their hive, and that must be scraped off so the frames can be separated. The beeswax, which contains some honey, bee parts, and other impurities, must be melted and filtered or strained. Most beeswax is gold or yellow but can also be in shades of orange, brown, etc. The color of the wax is in most part determined by the type of plants the bees collect nectar from. Beeswax has a delightful, light fragrance of honey, flower nectar and pollen. Beeswax makes superior, slow burning candles. Beeswax burns more beautifully than any other wax. It exudes a faint, natural fragrance of honey and pollen. When candles are made with the proper size of wicking, they are smokeless, dripless, and burn with a bright flame.

If you wonder why beeswax is so expensive, consider this: It has been estimated that bees must fly 150,000 miles to produce one pound of wax. Bees must eat about six pounds of honey to secrete a pound of wax. For every 100 pounds of honey a beekeeper harvests, only one to two pounds of beeswax are produced.

| **Moistening Vitamin E Cream** | **Antiseptic Balm** ( Use instead of antiseptic ointment, this is far superior! ) |
|---|---|
| 4 oz. sweet almond oil<br>1 oz. beeswax<br>2 oz. water<br>10 drops Vitamin E oil<br>10 drops lavender essential oil<br><br>Melt the oil and the wax in a double boiler, Remove from heat, add water, and stir thoroughly.<br><br>Add your Vitamin E, essential oil and stir continuously until cool. This cream is very moisturizing and emollient.<br><br>It is nice for rough, dry, or chapped complexions and should help promote healthy looking skin. After you have added the essential oil and the cream is still warm enough to pour, carefully pour it into Salve Jars or Metal Tins, we offer both below. | Ingredients:<br>2 ounces Beeswax<br>3 ounces Sweet Almond Oil<br>1 ounce Jojoba Oil<br>20 drops Wheatgerm Oil<br>20 drops Myrrh Essential Oil<br>20 drops Tea Tree Essential Oil<br>1 ounce of Colloidal Silver 10ppm<br>( Makes enough to fill 4 each 1 ounce salve jars or 1 ounce metal tins )<br><br>A rule of thumb is 2 parts oil to one part beeswax. Simply heat the Sweet Almond and Jojoba oil in a saucepan and add Beeswax. If you want a thin consistency ( such as a cream or Vaseline ) add only a little bit of Beeswax. Want it thicker like wax? Just add more Beeswax.<br>Allow the base to cool down to see what the consistency is like. If it's too thick, add more Sweet Almond oil and reheat, too thin?, add more Beeswax.<br>As the base is cooling add the essential oils to enhance the healing effect of the balm. These essential oils can be found in our Essential Oil List. After you have added the essential oil and the lip balm is still warm enough to pour, carefully pour it into Salve Jars or Metal Tins, we offer both below. |

## Herbal Salve

Make different Herbal Salves simply by changing/mixing different essential oils!
Ingredients:
2 ounces Beeswax
3 ounces Sweet Almond Oil
1 ounce Jojoba Oil
1/2 oz. Canola oil
40 drops total essential oil of your preference
½ Colloidal Silver ( Makes enough to fill 4 each 1 ounce salve jars or 1 ounce metal tins )

Simply heat the Sweet Almond, Canola oil and Jojoba oil in a saucepan and add Beeswax. If you want a thin consistency ( such as a cream or Vaseline ) add only a little bit of Beeswax. Want it thicker like wax? Just add more Beeswax.
Allow the base to cool down to see what the consistency is like. If it's too thick, add more Sweet Almond oil and reheat, too thin?, add more Beeswax.
As the base is cooling add the essential oils to enhance the healing effect of the balm. These essential oils can be found in our Essential Oil List.

After you have added the essential oil and the lip balm is still warm enough to pour, carefully pour it into Salve Jars or Metal Tins:

## REMEDIE HERBALS:

Use Bayleaf Essential oil for relieving rheumatism.
Use Bergamot Essential oil for colds, bronchitis systems, i.e. chest rub.
Use Caraway Essential oil for antiseptic quality.
Use Cardamon Essential oil for aphrodisiac quality. Use Clary Sage Essential oil for anti-ainflammatory, aphrodisiac and scalp problems. Use Cedar Essential oil for relieving Chronic anxiety and stress. Use Citronella Essential oil for making a insect repellent salve.
Use Eucalyptus Essential oil for chest rub, relieves congestion, eases breathing.
Use Frankincense Essential oil for asthma and other respiratory problems.
Use Gardenia Essential oil for chest rub, said to relieve flu conditions, fever, hypertension and palpitations. Use Juniper Essential oil for emotionally cleansing effect. Calms the nerves.
Use Orange Essential oil for a lighter body lotion, said to relax, relieve sexual apprehension, and is antiseptic and antibactericidal. Use Patchouli Essential oil for antiseptic, aphrodisiac qualities.
Use Rosemary Essential oil for relieving tired muscles.
Use Tea Tree Essential oil for Antiseptic, antifungal, antiviral qualities.

## Itch Relief Salve ( Good for posion ivy, posion oak )
1 pint Sweet Olive Oil
2 ounces Beeswax
1 tablespoon Chickweed Powder
1 tablespoon Comfrey Powder

Put chickweed and comfrey powder into sweet olive oil and simmer 3 hours. Strain and add beeswax. Pour into salve jars or tins.

## Vaseline Type Jelly
This makes a great vaseline type jelly.
1 ounce (weight) beeswax, 1/2 cup baby oil   Melt the beeswax in a microwave or a double boiler. Stir in the baby oil. Remove the mixture from the heat and stir until cool.

**Skin Cream** ( by Elaine White )

2 1/2 ounces (weight) beeswax
4 ounces (weight) lanolin
2/3 cup baby or mineral oil
3/4 cup water
1 teaspoon borax (sodium borate, CP)

Fragrant oil (optional)  - Melt the oil, lanolin and beeswax to 160 degrees F. Heat the borax and water in a separate container to 160 degrees F. Be sure the beeswax is melted and the borax is dissolved. Add the water mixture to the oil mixture while stirring.

When a white cream forms, stir slowly until the mixture cools to 100 degrees F. Pour the cream into small, wide-mouth jars.

**Pain Relief Salve**

1 tablespoon Chickweed powder
1 tablespoon Wormwood Powder
10 drops Tea Tree oil
2 pints Sweet Olive Oil
3 ounces Beeswax -  Mix together chickweed, wormwood powder, add the mixed herbs to sweet olive oil and simmer 3 hours. Strain and add beeswax and Tea Tree Oil. Pour into salve containers.

**Hand Cream**

2 ounces beeswax
1 cup sweet almond oil
1 cup water
10 drops essential oil (if desired, for fragrance)Heat beeswax and sweet almond oil until the wax melts. In another container, heat water until warm. Both mixtures should be warm, but not so hot as to be uncomfortable to the touch. Place warm water in a blender. Cover the blender, leaving open the small opening in the cover. With the blender running on high speed, slowly pour in the beeswax-oil mixture in a thin stream. When most of the oil has been added, the mixture should begin to thicken. At this point, add the essential oil. Continue to add oil and blend until the mixture is sufficiently thickened. Turn off the blender. You should have a thick cream. Spoon into salve jars or metal tins.

**Body Lotion**

This is a great recipe that does not spoil easily without the aid of refrigeration. It makes about 2 cups of lotion.

1 cup of aloe vera gel
1 teaspoon of lanolin 1 teaspoon of pure vitamin E oil
1/3 cup of coconut oil
1/2 ounce of beeswax
3/4 cup of almond oil
Up to 1 and 1/2 teapoons of essential oil of your choice or more to prolong scent

Place aloe vera gel, lanolin and vitamin E oil in a blender or food processor. Place coconut oil and beeswax in a 2 cup Pyrex measuring cup, microwave on high for 30 second and stir. Repeat in ten second blocks until fully melted. Stir in almond oil, reheating if necessary. Run blender at low to medium speed, then pour in melted oils in a thin stream. As the oils is blended in the cream will turn white and the blender's motor will begin to grind. As soon as you have a mayonnaise-like consistency, stop motor, add essential oils and pulse blend. do not over blend Transfer cream to glass jars while still warm because it thickens quickly.

## Guide Disclaimer and Use Information

While it has been our goal to share as much of our ideas and lab results freely with the world, we also have a legal copyright to this information. PRIDELABS and it's authors and researchers have spent hundreds of hours compiling this information from many un-copyrighted sources and from many hours of actual lab research and testing.

We understand that similar information may be available on other sites; we still hope to curb the dissemination of our latest experimental results to our competition and while they are all undergoing independent research and testing from many fellow researchers.

Unfortunately, some past researchers and customers have been electronically posting or sharing PRIDELABS proprietary information unlawfully via emails and posting or discussing our methods with other non-PRIDELABS Research Group Approved members.

We recently settled several lawsuits against one company owner and two past customers who have received this manual and its addendums who shared all or part of this licensed or proprietary methods/experiments with others, unlawfully and/or without written permission of Pride Labs or Pride Communications Co, LLC. PRIDELABS experiments and wording, (including diagrams) have special encoding that is we have the key to. Because of our key encoding, the courts ruled our copyright had been broken by the three past customers.

Most of these methods are purely informational and experimental; some have been tested by PRIDELABS while other's having not been tested, they are listed as 'informational uses' only.

The use of any method and or production experiment using any information contained herein is solely your own responsibility. The methods illustrated in this HVAC Experimenters Guide are not that of PRIDEALABS.US, nor will we publish any PRIDELABS.US proprietary production methods of the Colloidal Companies we distribute for, without their permission.

Random postings regarding any information contained herein are not allowed under our legal terms of disclosure and copyright, they should NOT be transmitted to and/or discussed on SILVER LISTS, GOLD LISTS, ESKIMO SILVER LISTS and other YAHOO GROUPS without permission of PRIDELABS.US or its authors.
When you receive this manual and addendums, you are bound by our Copyright and Disclosure terms of sale.

Please help us by not posting to these unauthorized internet groups.

You are only authorized to post, ask questions and discuss methods on the PRIIDELABS PRIVATE ONLINE RESEARCH GROUP ONLY.

**This INFORMATION contained in this manual is LEGALLY COPYRIGHTED and LICENSED TO PRIDELABS.US**

This manual and its associated diagrams and/or pictures are the SOLE property of PRIDELABS.US.

EVERY METHOD AND EXPERIMENT was ORIGINALLY DESIGNED, TESTED and

PUBLISHED by Pride Communications during March and April of 1998.

## EQUIPMENT DISCLAIMER

This information is intended for the use by advanced and experienced colloidal researchers only!

PRIDELABS.US, its owners, officers, employees or the authors of this Information cannot warranty, guaranty or promise that you will be able to effectively re-create ANY OF THE experiments contained in this manual.

YOUR EXPERIMENTS ARE YOURS ALONE, they do not represent PRIDELABS.US or any approved PRIDELABS production methods. We encourage you to get independent lab testing done on all your experiments to verify the usability and safety of any Colloidal minerals produced with any PRIDELABS.US power supply.

We cannot control your SLP effect, lab variables, your techniques or individual results, so legally, any liquids you make are YOURS ALONE and done so by your own individual methods. The outcome and testing results are yours alone. We will seek legal action against any Party or Lab which posts either favorable, non-favorable or inconclusive labs results and try to state they are actual PRIDELABS.US results.

Using High Voltage AC and DC power supplies can be potentially hazardous and because of this PRIDELABS.US takes no responsibility for your use of this kit. We also are not responsible for legal or medical complaints arising out of your use of this kit or of this information.  This guide is presented as an informational tool only and should be construed as such.


Thank you for reading this book, feel free to send your suggestions, experiments and methods and we will include them in the second printing and give you Credit for the submission, ideas and comments.

Send your correspondence to:

Mfp.pacific@gmail.com

Made in the USA
Lexington, KY
26 December 2012